DATA MAKES THE DIFFERENCE

DATA

MAKES THE DIFFERENCE

THE SMART NURSE'S HANDBOOK FOR USING DATA TO IMPROVE CARE

Kimberly S. Glassman, PhD, RN, NEA-BC

Peri Rosenfeld, PhD

American Nurses Association

Silver Spring, Maryland • 2015

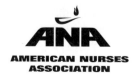

AMERICAN NURSES ASSOCIATION

American Nurses Association
8515 Georgia Avenue, Suite 400
Silver Spring, MD 20910-3492
1-800-274-4ANA
www.NursingWorld.org

Published by Nursesbooks.org
The Publishing Program of ANA
www.Nursesbooks.org/

The American Nurses Association (ANA) is the only full-service professional organization representing the interests of the nation's 3.1 million registered nurses through its constituent/state nurses associations and its organizational affiliates. The ANA advances the nursing profession by fostering high standards of nursing practice, promoting the rights of nurses in the workplace, projecting a positive and realistic view of nursing, and by lobbying the Congress and regulatory agencies on healthcare issues affecting nurses and the public.

Cataloging-in-Publication Data on file with the Library of Congress.

978-1-55810-611-6   SAN: 851-3481   1.5K   04/2015
First printing: April 2015

CONTENTS

PREFACE

This book represents a true collaboration between colleagues and contemporaries from different disciplines whose careers have been devoted to nurses, nursing and excellence in health care. Coming from different perspectives, we believe that the current focus on data, quality, safety and outcomes can shine a bright light on the roles nurses play in health care. Historical stereotypes of nurses as physician handmaidens (or sexy caregivers) have hindered the image of nurses as effective, independent decision-makers who stand at the helm of health care 24/7.

Dr. Glassman, who came up through the nursing ranks from staff nurse to Chief Nursing Officer at one of the nation's most prominent Academic Medical Centers, recognized the value of data-driven decision in transforming her leadership team from a group of RNs working in silos to a synergistic team of like-minded professionals. At NYU Langone Medical Center, Dr. Glassman leads a workforce of over 3000 RNs (from BSNs to MSNs to DNPs and PhDs) providing patient care in inpatient and ambulatory/community settings. Making the case for the financial, clinical and organizational benefits of nurses remains an ongoing dialogue as policy and payer decisions nip at the heels of all health care organizations. In an era of accountability and transparency, the imperative to demonstrate outcomes and assure evidence-based practices is an institutional priority for all providers. Nurses need to be active participants in these discussions and they must acquire the vocabulary and skill to "talk the talk" with colleagues at every levels of health care.

Dr. Rosenfeld, a health services researcher whose career led her to diverse organizations such as the National League for Nursing, NY State Council on Graduate Medical Education, NYU College of Nursing, New York Academy of Medicine and Visiting Nurses Service of New York is acutely aware that physicians, policy-makers, funders and foundation are simply ignorant of the far-reaching capabilities of nurses who possess unique skills and adhere to professional practices exclusively their own. Despite the enormity of the nursing workforce (over 3 million) and their increasingly sophisticated education and training, nurses are often not able to exploit available data for patient care decision-making or other purposes. With their focus on patient-centered care, nurses view each patient as individuals and may find it difficult to classify these individual characteristics into standardized categories, the hallmark of measurement and data-driven decision making. Our desire to help nurses increase their comfort level in generating, using and exploiting reliable data has been the primary motivator for us to write this book

The ultimate objective is to underscore nurse's contributions to the American health care system, which will remain hidden unless nurses demonstrate their value through empirical evidence, that is, research and data.

We sincerely acknowledge the contributions of Akiva Blander, Kathy Coichetti-Mazzeo, Halia Melnyk and Teresa Veneziano.

1

History, Background, and Introduction

Overview and Background

What do we mean by "quality" and how is it related to safety?

Over the past two to three decades, healthcare delivery and finance have changed dramatically due to the introduction of high tech innovations, closer financial scrutiny by private and public payers, and increased focus on patient and family care, to name a few. Arguably, the most powerful and transformative changes are associated with the growing influence of policies addressing the definition and measurement of quality and safety in healthcare. Early observers of the American healthcare system identified the existence of *iatrogenic effects* associated with surgical care, that is, preventable infections, adverse medication events, and any other complications associated with hospitalization (Illych, 1975). The perceived risk of hospital care remained under the radar until the 1990s when providers, policy-makers, and patient groups became more vocal about their concerns. Ultimately, the Institute of Medicine (IOM) launched a series of investigative studies to determine how widespread the safety and error risks were, and to identify the factors that facilitated the existence and growth of these serious problems. The pioneering work of the IOM studies, which will be summarized below, cannot be overstated. The findings of these seminal works prompted many important changes in the way health care is delivered and how providers practice. Hundreds of public and private groups grew out of the recommendations of these reports, some of which will be described in this volume.

One of the most enduring outcomes of the IOM reports have been their emphasis on accountability and the use of data to make accountability more transparent. The use of empirical data to monitor practice, track changes, establish long-term goals, and generally establish accountability at all levels of care, is undeniably a vital component in contemporary nursing practice.

Many registered nurses (RNs) are uncomfortable with discussions of data, measures, and statistics. RNs often say, "I'm not good with numbers" or "I hated my statistics class," though they are competent at dosing, using assessment tools, and other practices that require knowledge of measurement and data. Nurses may not realize that the data used for many quality and safety purposes within their practice setting come directly from their daily documentation of the patient care they provide.

Several years ago, one of us gave a workshop at our workplace for RNs on reading and interpreting data on scorecards. Among the topics discussed was delving deeply into data from the institutional level to the unit level and from the unit level to the individual RN level. A series of sample illustrations were provided, and the take-away message was that, in an era of accountability, it was possible to identify those services, units, or individual practitioners whose performance did not meet the expected or desired goal for the organization. One RN asked the question on everyone's mind: "Where did you get all the data for all those charts and tables?" The answer: From you! A gasp of disbelief was heard in the room. It is worth repeating: When an RN digitally enters data on patient care and nursing practices on their unit, regardless of the information technology system, they are supplying information that is then aggregated, manipulated, and reported for manifold purposes internal and external to the organization itself.

Nurses are vital to our search for and understanding of quality and safety, not only because of their competence and devotion to excellent patient care, but also because they are the creators of the data necessary to measure nurses' contributions to patients and organizational outcomes in their workplaces. One goal of this book is to help RNs understand their important contributions to ensuring accurate and meaningful quality and safety data that reflects the overall contributions of RNs to sustaining and improving the American healthcare system.

The Institute of Medicine Reports: Pioneering Work on Quality and Safety in Health Care

The Institute of Medicine (IOM) issued four seminal reports that represent the genesis of the quality and safety movements in health care.

To Err is Human (1999)

To Err is Human: Building a Safer Health Care System, released in 1999, defined medical errors as "either a failure of a planned action as intended, or using the wrong means to achieve an aim" and estimated that medical errors have killed between 44,000 and 98,000 people, and has cost 17 or 29 billion dollars per year in additional health care required, lost productivity, and disability, as well as other negative outcomes (IOM, 1999). The report concluded that the "nation's epidemic of medical errors" is not the result of "bad apples," but rather the result of faulty systems, processes, and conditions that lead to mistakes despite good intentions. The lack of incentives among accrediting bodies and payers to focus on issues of quality and safety contributes to these negative outcomes.

Based on its exhaustive research on the causes of and contributors to medical errors, the report recommends a four-tiered strategy for improvement (IOM, 1999; Sloan, 2008):

- Establish a national focus to create tools and protocols that enhance the knowledge base about safety through the creation of the Center for Patient Safety, housed with the Department of Health and Human Services' (DHHS) Agency for Healthcare Research and Quality (AHRQ), to set national safety goals and track progress; develop a research agenda; and other activities to raise awareness among consumers and providers regarding safety improvement.

- Learn from errors through a nationwide public mandatory reporting system and encourage healthcare organizations, beginning with hospitals, to develop voluntary reporting systems. State governments should be required to collect standardized information about medical events that result in injury or death. Voluntary reporting systems can focus on a wide range of errors, particularly those that inflict minimal harm, and help detect weaknesses in the system that, if fixed, can prevent more serious harm.

- Raise performance standards and expectations for improvement through oversight organizations, professional groups, and group healthcare purchasers. Performance standards can be set through regulatory mechanisms, such as licensing, certification, and accreditation, which can define minimum performance levels for health professionals and their organizations, as well as the tools (drugs and devices) they use. Professional associations, accrediting bodies, and larger purchasers of health care can also set standards, provide incentives, and raise awareness to reduce errors, and improve safety.

- Create a culture of safety within healthcare organizations by implementing safety systems to ensure safe practices at the delivery level. This can be accomplished by incorporating safety principles, such as designing jobs and conditions with safety in mind, standardizing equipment and processes, and enabling providers to avoid relying on memory to deliver care.

The report also identified several principles for designing safer institutions, including the presence of healthcare leadership committed to quality and safety, increased use of practice guidelines and standards to improve care rather than reliance on memory, effective teamwork, creation of systems that help plan for the unexpected, and creating a blame-free environment where quality and safety can be discussed freely.

To be sure, not all of the recommendations of the IOM report have been fully implemented (Robert Wood Johnson, 2009; Wachter, 2010; Clancy, 2009). Nonetheless, the publication of *To Err is Human* is considered a landmark report that has catalyzed dramatic changes in the way hospitals and other healthcare organizations monitor their performance regarding quality and safety. The report's insistence on public and voluntary reporting led to the creation and expansion of governmental and private initiatives to develop and widely disseminate standardized definitions of quality and safety, uniform data collection tools and measures, as well as widely accepted processes for measuring quality and strategies for its improvement.

Crossing the Quality Chasm (2001)

Two years after *To Err is Human*, the Institute of Medicine released *Crossing the Quality Chasm: A New Health System for the 21st Century* (IOM, 2001a), which focused more broadly on how the healthcare system can be reinvented to foster innovation and improve the delivery of care. Acknowledging the ever-increasing complexity and fragmented nature of services located in silos across the healthcare delivery system, the report calls for far-reaching changes to improve provider performance and patient outcomes.

The report calls for all healthcare groups (professionals, policymakers, purchasers of care, regulators, managers, boards, consumers, etc.) to commit to a national statement of purpose for the healthcare system as a whole, by accepting an explicit objective to reduce harm and the burden of illness as well as to improve the health and well-being of all people (Chassin, 2002). The report outlines six aims to provide safer, more reliable, and more responsive care, as well as care that is more integrated and more accessible. Together these changes would enable healthcare providers to better do their jobs (Wakefield, 2008). These aims include being:

1. **Safe**—Avoid injuries to patients and healthcare providers
2. **Effective**—Provide services based on scientific knowledge
3. **Patient-centered**—Provide care that is respectful and responsive to individual preferences, needs, and values
4. **Timely**—Reduce wait times and harmful delays for caregivers and patients
5. **Efficient**—Avoid waste of equipment, supplies, ideas, or energy
6. **Equitable**—Provide quality care independent of personal characteristics, such as race, ethnicity, and sexual orientation

These six aims for high-quality care are critical to fostering a culture of quality in healthcare organizations. Since the publication of *Crossing the Quality Chasm*, there has been a great deal of effort made to define and measure these six aims to ensure data is standardized across a variety of healthcare settings (Wakefield, 2008). A wide range of public and private organizations are engaged in setting standards in each of these areas. Most notable is Patient Centered Outcomes Research Institute (PCORI), an AHRQ agency devoted to supporting research on increasing our understanding of patient and caregiver engagement outcomes.

Furthermore, *Crossing the Quality Chasm* proposed four areas within the healthcare environment to be addressed:

- **Applying evidence to healthcare delivery**: The report recommends that DHHS establish a comprehensive program to make scientific evidence more useful and accessible to clinicians and patients alike. Leadership from the private sector must be involved in all stages of this effort to ensure applicability and acceptability to clinicians and patients, focusing on priority conditions. Efforts should include: analysis of evidence, delineation of practice guidelines, identification of best practices, dissemination of evidence to professionals, development of support tools in applying evidence and making decisions, establishment of goals for improvement in processes and outcomes, and development of measures to assess quality of care.

- **Using information technology:** Central to the information technology applications is the automation of patient-specific clinical information. Current information is poorly organized or difficult to access. Also, patients should be able to communicate via email with professionals. Finally, automated systems for ordering medication are recommended to reduce errors in prescription and dosage and should include reminders for patients and clinicians.

- **Implications for workforce:** Implicit in the recommendations of *Crossing the Quality Chasm* is the need to prepare the workforce to work in a revamped healthcare system. Nurses and other providers need training that emphasizes interdisciplinary, evidence-based care, and that accounts for the importance of data in tracking practice and patient trends for regulation and accreditation purposes.

- **Align payment policies to quality outcomes:** Incentives to address quality improvements, can be adopted in varying degrees by government payers (Medicare and Medicaid) and insurance companies through pay for performance (P4P) programs. These topics will be discussed in greater detail in later chapters.

The report set forth "10 Rules of Health Care Design" (see Sidebar 1.1) which, when first published in 2001, were considered revolutionary. Yet today, they are integral parts of how we provide care in the contemporary healthcare system, specifically nursing care. Undoubtedly, many of these rules are still works in progress, yet their attainment is at the very core of nursing practice.

Keeping Patients Safe: Transforming the Work Environment of Nurses (2003)

These two IOM reports led to extensive dialogue among government and private stakeholders regarding strategies and approaches to increase the quality and safety of health care in the American healthcare system, which led to the realization of the key role of nurses in patient safety, particularly in hospitals. Thus, the AHRQ asked the IOM to conduct a study to examine the key aspects of the nursing work environment that likely have an impact on patient safety, and discover potential improvements in healthcare working conditions that would likely increase patient safety (Page, 2008).

IOM was further directed to study the impact of workplace environment, systems, and staffing policies that may influence nurses' ability to provide high-quality, safe care. The study concluded that the typical

SIDEBAR 1.1

TEN RULES OF HEALTHCARE DESIGN: CROSSING THE QUALITY CHASM

1. Care is based on continuous healing relationships: patients should receive care at any time and in many forms, not only face-to-face visits.

2. Care is customized according to patient needs and values rather than provider preference: the system should meet the most common needs but should also be able to respond to patient choices and preferences.

3. The patient is the source of control: they should be given the opportunity and information to exercise however much control over care decisions they want.

4. Knowledge is shared and information flows freely: patients should have unfettered access to their own information, as well as to clinical information. Clinicians and patients should share information and communicate effectively.

5. Decision-making is evidence-based: care is based on the best available scientific knowledge and should not vary illogically depending on place or person.

6. Safety is a system property: patients should be safe from injury caused by the system. Reducing risk and ensuring safety requires greater attention to prevention and error mitigation systems.

7. Transparency is necessary: information should be made available to patients that enables them to make informed decisions, including information describing the system's performance in the areas of safety, evidence-based practice, and patient satisfaction.

8. Needs are anticipated: the system should anticipate needs of patients, rather than simply reacting to issues that arise

9. Waste is continually decreased: there should not be any waste of resources or patient time

10. Cooperation among clinicians is a priority: clinicians and institutions should collaborate and communicate for an exchange of information and coordination of care.

Source: IOM 2001a

work environment of nurses poses many serious threats to patient safety, which are found in all four of the basic components of organizations—organizational management practices, workforce deployment practices, work design, and organizational culture. The report recommended dramatic changes in nurses' work environment that would facilitate the reduction of medical errors and other adverse events.

The recommendations in *Keeping Patients Safe* are built upon the recommendations from the two prior IOM reports: *To Err Is Human: Building a Safer Health System* (1999) and *Crossing the Quality Chasm: A New Health System for the 21st Century* (2001a). The recommendations provided a blueprint that healthcare organizations could use to create a culture of safety and to address work design to ensure safer environments. The report focused a much-needed spotlight on the importance of ensuring adequate nursing staff, curbing unprofessional and disruptive behavior, and increasing the roles and responsibilities of nurse leadership (Page, 2008). *Keeping Patients Safe* emphasized the critical need for timely, reliable data on key nursing practices associated with patient outcomes. The recognition that the quality of the nursing workforce and nursing practice has a direct impact on patient outcomes is one of the enduring legacies of this landmark report. It sent a clarion call to all healthcare organizations to consistently monitor nursing-related quality and safety indicators and pursue continuous quality improvement (Kurtzman, Fauteaux, 2014).

Performance evaluations can range from on-going quality assessment processes to formal evaluations of specific initiatives. Inherent in all discussions of the impact of practices and processes on patient safety and other care delivery outcomes, however, is the need for continuous assessment of performance and impact, and the essence of these assessments is collection, analysis, and reporting of standardized data over time and across organizations.

Keeping Patients Safe inspired the creation of several initiatives that have had an enduring impact on assessing nursing practices and quality outcomes. For example, Transforming Care at the Bedside (TCAB) is a Robert Wood Johnson Foundation Institute for Healthcare Improvement (RWJF IHI) program designed to improve care by empowering nurses to address certain quality and safety issues on their units, instead of relying on traditional top–down approaches, and has resulted in measurable improvements in bedside care (Naylor, Lustig, Kelly, Melichor, &

Pauly, 2013; Robert Wood Johnson, 2009). Nurse engagement in quality improvement is now integral to most hospitals.

In addition, the National Database on Nursing Quality Indicators (NDNQI) allows hospitals to chart their performance on quality and practice metrics and compare them to other healthcare organizations. NDNQI is a major resource to measure quality, safety, and patient outcomes (http://www.nursingquality.org/). The National Quality Forum (NQF) brings together a wide range of stakeholders to create consensus on standard measures of quality. Finally, credentialing organizations, such as The Joint Commission (TJC), evaluate healthcare organizations on patient care and organizational functions essential to safe and high-quality care. Through its accreditation processes, TJC promotes standardized data collection, reporting, and benchmarking. Similarly, the Magnet Accreditation Program®, which recognizes organizations that employ and retain top nursing talent, also requires evidence of highly effective nurse workplaces. More detailed discussions of some of these initiatives will be presented in later chapters.

The Future of Nursing (2010)

A great deal of research and analyses were undertaken subsequent to the release of *Keeping Patients Safe* in order to fully understand the influence of the nursing workforce, nursing practices, and workplace policies on quality, safety, and patient outcomes. It became clear that a number of barriers prevented nurses from being able to respond effectively to rapidly changing healthcare settings and an evolving healthcare system. These barriers must be surmounted in order to ensure that nurses are well-positioned to lead change and advance health care. Thus, the IOM commissioned a report to offer recommendations for an action-oriented blueprint to allow nurses to be change agents and spearhead initiatives that would improve practices, policies, and outcomes. This report, titled *The Future of Nursing: Leading Change, Advancing Health*, provides a thorough analysis of the nursing workforce and discussion of how nurses are key players in providing high-quality patient care in all settings and at all stages of care. The report contains recommendations designed to reduce existing barriers that impede nurses, while also increasing opportunities for nurses to take advantage of their knowledge and talents to make the biggest impact on care.

The report advances four key areas to ensure the future of nursing:

1. Nurses should practice to the full extent of their education and training.
2. Nurses should achieve higher levels of education and training through an improved education system that promotes seamless academic progression.
3. Nurses should be full partners with physicians and other professionals in redesigning health care in the United States. This includes collaborative efforts at identifying problems and areas of system waste, devising improvement plans, tracking improvement, and making necessary adjustments to realize goals.
4. Effective workforce planning and policymaking requires better data collection and an improved information infrastructure. In addition, planning for changes in the nursing workforce requires comprehensive data on types and numbers of health professionals.

Together, these four themes underscore the regrettable reality that nurses are often unable to practice at the levels for which they were educated and—due to many organizational, political, and other factors—are often not considered full partners with physicians in tackling quality and safety issues. This must change if healthcare organizations are serious about providing the highest quality patient care possible. Nurses must be actively engaged in designing improvement plans, identifying feasible measures, and tracking quality data to accumulate the evidence to support that targets are being met and positive patient outcomes are being realized (Spetz, Bates, Chu, Lin, Fishman & Melichor, 2013). While the primary focus of this report has been on hospitals, the IOM has issued separate papers on nursing in long-term care settings (IOM, 2001b).

Other Seminal Reports: Carnegie Study on Nursing Education
There are multiple educational pathways into the nursing profession, and a long-standing debate exists as to the ideal educational preparation for RNs. Nurses today can obtain an RN license through several educational routes: getting an associate degree through community colleges, an RN diploma through a hospital-based school of nursing, a baccalaureate degree in a four-year college, or the recent accelerated programs, which require a BA in another discipline and offer the BS in nursing in 15–18 months, as well as generic master's degree programs.

As nursing care has become increasingly more complex and dependent on technological innovation, nursing leaders have proposed that the baccalaureate degree is the more appropriate educational preparation to practice nursing (AONE, 2005). Supported by a resolution in the 2008 American Nurses Association (ANA) House of Delegates, many states are now considering legislation to require a baccalaureate degree in nursing for RN licensure and would allow RNs with other degrees to obtain their BS degrees in a designated amount of time, such as ten years for New Jersey, New York, and Ohio (AACN, 2014; ANA, 2011, Hilton, 2012; New York State Assembly, 2015–2016 General Assembly, A03945/S02145; https://legiscan.com/NY/bill/A03945/2015).

Nurses, the largest group of healthcare providers, spend the most time with hospitalized patients, provide the majority of home care, and arguably have the most influence on patient outcomes. Nurses today must manage complex technology while supporting the significant needs of hospitalized patients and families. Studies note the importance of both nurses' educational preparation and nurse staffing on improved patient outcomes (Needleman et al., 2011; Kovner, 1998; Aiken, 2011). The convergence of increasing complexity in our healthcare system with anticipated nursing and faculty shortages prompted the Carnegie Foundation to undertake a review of the state of nursing education in the United States (Benner, 1982; Benner, Sutphen, Leonard, & Day, 2009). Benner's findings revealed that the current system of educating nurses was inadequate to meet the increasingly complex needs of patients, especially as the U.S. population ages. The authors noted the need to increase the quality and delivery of education to nurses to meet the needs of the public in all care settings.

The call for a Bachelor of Science in Nursing (BSN) prepared nursing workforce is stymied by anticipated shortages among faculty of higher education (Allan & Aldebron, 2008; NACNEP, 2010). Nonetheless, the Carnegie report calls for a transformation of nursing education to advance knowledge, judgment, skills, and ethical standards for those who aspire to enter the nursing profession, all important elements of BSN education (Benner, Sutphen, Leonard, & Day, 2009). The report examined various programs of nursing pre-licensure preparation through surveys, observations, and interviews with faculty and students in a representative sample of varied programs. The major findings were:

- U.S. nursing programs are very effective in forming professional identity and promoting ethical behavior,

- Clinical practice assignments provide powerful learning experiences, especially in those programs where educators integrate clinical and classroom teaching,

- U.S. nursing programs are not generally effective in teaching nursing science, natural sciences, social sciences, technology, and humanities, and

- The challenges are presented as a call to action by all sectors of the profession: Practicing education and policy supports the advancement of the nursing profession in leading the changes to the healthcare delivery system.

Quality and Safety Education for Nurses (QSEN)

In 2003, confronted by the Institute of Medicine Health Professions Education report (IOM, 2003), more attention was focused on the role of nurses in promoting high-quality patient-centered care as members of an interdisciplinary team, using evidence-based practice, quality improvement techniques, and informatics at the bedside. In order to meet that demand, and to highlight the importance of the nursing profession in care delivery, nursing educators and leaders met to define the qualities and competencies needed for nurses to be masters of quality and safety. Thus, the Quality and Safety Education for Nurses (QSEN), funded by RWJF, was developed to design the future of nursing education to meet these demands (Cronenwett, 2012; Cronenwett, Sherwood, & Gelmon, 2009). An advisory board of thought-leaders in nursing and health care was formed to review the IOM competencies, which subsequently were adapted for all registered nurses. In a process that included multiple reviews of nursing competencies by academies, clinicians, and administrators, QSEN identified six competencies that emphasized quality and safety in nursing. The QSEN competencies are as follows:

1. **Patient-centered:** Recognize the patient or designee as the source of control and a full partner in providing compassionate and coordinated care based on respect for the patient's preferences, values, and needs.

2. **Teamwork and collaboration:** Function effectively within nursing and inter-professional teams, fostering open communication, mutual respect, and shared decision-making to achieve quality patient care.

3. **Evidence-based practice:** Integrate the best, most scientifically robust, current evidence with clinical expertise, patient/family preferences, and values for delivery of optimal health care.

4. **Quality improvement:** Use data to monitor the outcomes of care processes and use improvement methods to design and test changes to continuously improve the quality and safety of healthcare systems.

5. **Safety:** Minimize the risk of harm to patients and providers through both system design and individual performance.

6. **Informatics:** Use information technology to communicate, manage knowledge, mitigate error, and support decision-making.

The knowledge, skills, and attitudes that are reflective of these competencies can be found at the QSEN website (www.qsen.org).

Nurses are Key to Quality

Strength in Numbers

The persistent focus on nurse's contributions to quality and safety is predicated on a simple fact: nurses are ubiquitous. They are present in every part of healthcare delivery. Several data sources exist that estimate the size of the nursing workforce. According to the last DHHS Sample Survey of Registered Nurses conducted in 2008, there were an estimated 3,063,162 licensed registered nurses living in the United States, (U.S. DHHS, 2010). A very large percentage of licensed RNs (84.8%) were employed in nursing positions (n = 2,596,599).

In the absence of a current full RN Sample Survey, the Health Resources and Services Administration released a report in 2014 projecting national and state supply and demand for RNs from 2012–2025. The projection model concluded that approximately 2.9 million RNs were active in the workforce in 2012 and the supply is expected to continue growing for the foreseeable future (U.S. DHHS, 2014).

Comparable data on physicians, collected in 2006, found an estimated 817,500 medical (MD) and osteopathic (OD) physicians in the United States, less than 1/3 the number of RNs (U.S. DHHS, 2006).

The Bureau of Labor Statistics Occupational Employment Statistics Survey (2013) is another well-known source of data on the nursing workforce. According to these data, released in 2013, a majority of employed RNs (62%) reported that they worked in general medical/surgical, psychiatric, or other specialty hospitals. Ambulatory care is another common employment setting, containing almost 13% of employed RNs. Approximately 7% of employed RNs work in long-term care facilities. Due to the prevalence of RNs in hospitals, this volume will often focus on quality issues and data as they pertain to acute care settings. Additional discussions of the use of quality and safety data in other settings will be included in various sections.

There have been impressive advances in quality and safety in hospital care since the release of *To Err Is Human*, though additional improvements are undoubtedly needed. Somewhat slower progress has been made in long-term care and home care, though recent innovations in healthcare payment systems such as Accountable Care Organizations and Integrated Health Care Systems have created much-needed focus on quality in non-hospital settings.

Nurses are the Eyes and Ears of Health Care

Registered nurses provide around-the-clock care in hospitals and thus, can monitor and detect changes in a patient's condition quickly. Registered nurses provide the majority of health care in hospitals, and patients rely on their astute assessment and observational ability to ensure quality and safety at the bedside (Mitchell, 2008). While many hospitals now have critical care physicians, or intensivists, in hospitals 24/7, the availability and proximity of RNs to patients makes nurses the critical nexus between patients and physicians—simply, doctors respond to a patient's bedside because they were called by a nurse. Due to their intimate knowledge of organizational structures and processes, nurses are accurate assessors of the overall quality of care provided by their institutions. A study by McHugh and Witkoski Stimpfel (2012) found that nurses' assessments of the quality of care in their workplace aligned well with quality and safety data reported to regulatory agencies. In other words, RNs are astute observers of the quality of the care provided by their institutions.

Nurses' Impact on Quality

The impact of nurses on the quality of care delivered in hospitals is also informed by the nurse-sensitive outcomes, such as number of falls, number of hospital-acquired pressure ulcers, number of hospital-acquired infections, medication errors, and other measures of hospital-acquired conditions or HACs (Frith et al., 2010; Haberfelde, Bedecarre & Buffum, 2005; Lucero, Lake & Aiken, 2010).

Organization of the Book

This chapter has presented a historical and conceptual history of the emergence of the quality and safety movement in nursing and health care. The measuring of quality and outcomes, a relatively new phenomenon, is now integral to our practices.

Chapter 2 will examine a range of issues related to our understanding of data—how it is defined, how it is collected, who decides what quality is, and what are the main types of data relevant to quality and nursing.

Chapter 3 examines why quality data is so important in contemporary nursing practice and how RNs at every level of practice must understand its value and benefit to patient care.

Chapter 4 looks toward the future of quality data—how the advent of electronic health records, (EHRs) will dramatically change how data is collected and used in the future. This chapter also contains a discussion of the power of analytic models to help predict which patients are at risk for different adverse events (readmissions, infections, falls, etc.) and the investment states are making to encourage sharing data across institutions (e.g., HEAL NY).

Chapter 5 provides case studies and other illustrations of quality data. In addition, the final chapter will summarize the key points covered in the book from the perspective of a CNO (chief nursing officer) of an academic medical center.

2

Quality Data: Definitions, Measures, and Metrics

This chapter will examine a range of issues related to our understanding of data—how it is defined, how it is collected, who decides what quality is, and what the main types of data relevant to quality and nursing are.

What is Quality Data and Quality Measurement?

Healthcare providers are surrounded by many types of data that come from multiple sources. Most obviously, providers deal with clinical data regarding their patients, which includes everything collected on admission and discharge assessments; services rendered during hospitalization of episode of care; medications and devices; manifold assessment and risk tools; results of tests; and so on. In addition to clinical data, providers also collect and utilize other patient-level data such as demographic and household characteristics, admission and discharge dates, and languages spoken, to name a few. Providers also work with administrative data such as types of insurance, history of appointments, use of other providers, etc. Each of these types of data is typically represented as a numerical value that expresses the meaning of the information (Rosenfeld, 2006). For example, thermometers measure temperature and specific readings have particular meanings regarding the health of the patient. Other common measures are time (using a clock), weight (scale), and blood pressure. These types of data are called string or continuous data.

String/continuous data can be further characterized as *interval* or *ordinal*. Ordinal data is best understood in terms of subjective attitudinal scales where choices (also known as values) are numbers that correspond with responses such as strongly agree (1), agree (2), neither agree nor disagree (3), disagree (4), or strongly disagree (5). Taking this example further, the difference between a response of 2 (agree) and a response of 4 (disagree) does not tell us exactly how different the respondents feel, but we get the sense that there is some level of difference between the two respondents. In the case of interval data, the different values are equidistant from one another so that we can be sure of how much the values differ. One illustration is a ruler. Each inch is exactly the same length as other inches; if a child grew 3 inches in a year, we understand that each of the 3 inches the child grew is equivalent to the 3 inches that other children grew during the same time.

Another type of numerical data may reflect simple "yes/no" or "male/female" categories and do not have any real meaning beyond the number assigned. Survey questions and checklists are common examples of these types of *categorical* data. Understanding the different types of numerical data is essential to monitoring quality and safety.

In short, healthcare providers have access to astounding amounts of *quantitative* data that can be combined in different ways to allow the user to better understand the effectiveness of care on patient outcomes. Each numerical data point, whether temperature or an affirmative response to a question, is considered an *observation*. The technical term for observable information is *empirical* data. The provider's ability to observe and record patient or other types of observations in numerical form is the cornerstone of *measurement*. The term *metric* represents a formula or combination of measures that measure change over time, such as length of stay or number of hospitalizations.

Qualitative data includes non-numerical information that is collected in written or descriptive form. Commonly used forms of qualitative data include information gathered through interviews, focus groups, direct observation, and analysis of written documents. Qualitative data has important benefits for clinical practice, research, and policy, particularly in instances when providers want to understand a specific phenomenon such as the experiences of patients with end-of-life decision-making or how immigrants learn about the American healthcare system. Qualitative data has less of a direct role in monitoring and assessing healthcare quality and safety. Frequently, however, qualitative data is systematically transformed into numerical values to allow for quantitative analysis.

It is important to make the distinction between primary and secondary data collection and analysis because:

- Primary data is information collected first-hand by an individual or researcher to study a topic they want to understand; the data is new in that it comes directly from the researchers and the participants or documents they examine.
- Secondary data analysis is re-examining data that has already been collected for another purpose in order to answer specific questions. Analysis of administrative data and patient-level data for quality and safety purposes is a form of secondary analysis.

The rest of this chapter will focus on how nursing uses quality measures and metrics to demonstrate their effectiveness in achieving patient and other outcomes.

Donabedian: A Useful Model for Thinking About Types of Data and the People Who Use Data for Nursing Practice

Avedis Donabedian, a physician, theorized that all health systems consist of environment (structure), process, and outcomes (*Donabedian, 1966*). The Donabedian model is one of the most widely-used in health services research. Structure, or environment, measures include staff, space, and equipment. Some commonly used structural measures are: number of staff on a unit; nurse educational level and skill mix; number of registered professional nurses or other providers; number of beds; and payers of healthcare services. Process measures reflect the way care is organized and delivered, such as heart failure discharge instructions; smoking cessation patient education; timeliness of antibiotics in sepsis; documentation of safety guidelines; and medication reconciliation at discharge. These measures give us information about how timely and completely our care is delivered. Outcome measures are results of the delivered care, and they are measured with a range of primarily quantitative outputs. Mortality is the most common outcome measure. Readmission within 30 days, a new publicly reported quality measure by CMS, is another outcome measure that suggests that there were deficiencies in the transitional care and community management of a patient or group of patients.

Comparing Apples to Apples: Standardized Definitions and Shared Metrics Related to Quality

The notion of metrics (also termed *measurements*) is borrowed from other fields such as business and finance, where the term describes a set of measurements to quantify results or outcomes. Thus, nursing metrics are ways of measuring the quality of nursing care and include indicators that measure nurse-delivered outcomes and patient experiences. With the increased interest in nursing quality in recent years by policy-makers and managers, measuring outcomes through metrics has been the subject of greater interest (Foulkes, 2011).

A critical aspect of measurement and metrics is the use of standard definitions of the phenomenon being observed, regardless of whether the object being observed is clinical, administrative, or financial (Rosenfeld, 2006; Shekelle, 2013). This means that clinicians typically use the same scale on their thermometers (e.g., Fahrenheit or Celsius) rather than idiosyncratic scales that are unique to a small group of practitioners. In addition, the use of standard timeframes (monthly, quarterly, year-to-date, etc.) makes it possible to monitor practices across time intervals that are reasonable and useful for decision-making. In summary, the use of standardized definitions and standardized tools and scales are critical to measurement because they:

- Promote objectivity by reducing the guesswork when making decisions,
- Permit comparisons across teams/units, regions, and other similar agencies throughout the nation (e.g., Academic Medical Centers, Children's Hospitals, Certified Home Health Agencies, etc.),
- Allow tracking of data over time,
- Provide empirical (observed) evidence of the outcomes of practices,
- Allow quantification of our processes and outcomes and the use of statistical analysis of large amounts of information, and
- Improve reliability of data.

Each healthcare professional group has its own mission, principles, tenets, and objectives. As such, certain indicators measure nursing's contribution to safety, effectiveness, and compassion, reflecting the unique contributions of nurses to patient care. Measures of the contributions of physicians or other providers may be vastly different. Ideally, indicators of quality nursing care should be: (i) measurable using existing data; (ii) evidence-based and linked to important outcomes; (iii) able to inform action plans; (iv) sensitive to nursing and its variability and recognized as the responsibility of the nursing staff; (v) accepted as important to nurses, managers, and consumers; (vi) risk-adjusted to compare performance across settings; (vii) something that minimizes the risk of "perverse incentive," where improving on the indicator detracts from overall actual performance and quality (Griffiths et al., 2008).

Types of Data and Measures of Nursing Quality

Data on quality come in many different forms and have many different purposes:

- Quality data for regulatory compliance
- Data for assessing achievement of performance targets
- Data to support accreditation (TJC/Magnet)
- Data to inform improvement (Lean Six Sigma)
- Predictive models in quality and safety improvement
- Data collected for research purposes

In this section, we will outline the primary types of data collection activities involving quality measures and metrics.

Quality Data for Regulatory Compliance

Findings from the IOM reports discussed in Chapter 1 lead to calls for public/consumer access to data on the outcomes of healthcare services to inform their healthcare decisions. Consumer access to outcomes can result in greater transparency and accountability of providers and healthcare organizations. Mortality rates were among the first publicly reported outcomes for hospitals and many more indicators are now publicly available.

Centers for Medicare and Medicaid Services

Hospitals, home care agencies, and other healthcare settings are required to report quality and safety data to demonstrate compliance to regulatory requirements. Much of this type of data is called "public reporting", since various governmental bodies require their systematic collection as part of public reimbursement (Lansky, 2012; Smith, 2013). The Centers for

Medicare and Medicaid Services (CMS) is a federal agency under the U.S. DHHS that administers Medicare and, in cooperation with state governments, Medicaid. It is also involved in the administration of Health Information Protection (HIPAA), quality standards in nursing homes, clinical laboratory quality standards, and Healthcare.gov. Healthcare organizations that receive Medicaid or Medicare funding are required to provide data on quality process and outcome measures. One of the most important purposes of these data is to provide consumers with information on how well different healthcare organizations perform on different quality measures.

Hospital Compare (see http://www.medicare.gov/hospitalcompare/about/what-is-HOS.html), created through the efforts of Medicare and the Hospital Quality Alliance (HQA), is a consumer-oriented website that provides information on how well hospitals provide recommended care to their patients. This information can help consumers make informed decisions about health care. Hospital Compare allows consumers to select multiple hospitals and directly compare performance measurement information related to heart attacks, heart failure, pneumonia, surgery, and other conditions. The Hospital Quality Alliance (HQA): Improving Care through Information was created in December 2002. In 2005, the first set of 10 core process of care measures were displayed on such topics as heart attacks, heart failure, pneumonia, and surgical care. Additional measures have been added over time.

It is noteworthy that CMS requires public reporting on patient experience as one of its key outcome measures. CMS, along with the AHRQ, developed the Hospital Consumer Assessment of Healthcare Providers and Systems (HCAHPS) Survey, also known as Hospital CAHPS®, to provide a standardized survey instrument and data collection methodology for measuring patients' perspectives on hospital care. The HCAHPS Survey is administered to a random sample of patients continuously throughout the year. CMS cleans, adjusts, and analyzes the data, then publicly reports the results.

Hospital Compare is one example of public reporting of quality data. Comparable public reporting is available for home care (see Sidebar 2.1 for more details), nursing homes, and other healthcare services. These data are used by more than just consumers and regulators. Individual healthcare organizations may use these data to identify areas of service or care that could be improved and subsequently design quality improvement initiatives.

SIDEBAR 2.1

HOSPITAL COMPARE

Make Informed Decisions about Health Care

Access the Hospital Compare Web site at www.hospitalcompare.hhs.gov. The data are organized by:

- Timely and effective care

- Readmissions, complications, and deaths

- Use of medical imaging

- Linking quality to payment

- Medicare volume

In addition, Hospital Compare also reports the results of the Hospital Consumer Assessment of Health Care Providers and Systems (HCAHPS) patient surveys in the following areas:

- Hospital nurse communication

- Doctor communication

- Responsiveness of hospital staff

- Pain management

- Communication about medicines

- Discharge information

- Cleanliness of hospital environment

- Quietness of hospital environment

- Overall rating of hospital

- Willingness to recommend hospital

Source: Center for Medicare & Medicaid Services (CMS). Survey of patients' experiences (www.medicare.gov.hospital compare/data/overview.html)

The AHRQ issued a report in 2012 to examine the effectiveness of public reporting of healthcare quality information as a quality improvement strategy (AHRQ, 2012). The report concluded that publicly reported quality measures are more likely to influence healthcare provider behaviors and less likely to have influence on consumer decision-making than originally expected. Analyses of Hospital Compare (and the other Compare sites) suggest that small numbers of consumers have used these websites (Ryan, Nallamothu, & Dimick, 2012; Werner & Bradlow, 2010). A recent report argues that increasing interest in public reporting websites must "recognize that consumers want information relevant to them—not necessarily what experts think they want," and that, rather than trying to lure consumers to government websites, information should be easily accessible through integration into more popular websites and technological innovations such as apps (Ryan et al., 2012).

National Patient Safety Goals

Quality and safety are treated almost as synonyms in health care (Mitchell, 2008). Yet, as described in Chapter 1, there are conceptual differences: safety is typically understood as the prevention or reduction of harm, a primary principle in health care reflected in the Hippocratic Oath. Quality is the degree to which practices meet professionally defined standards and cover more abstract concepts such as patient centeredness or symptom management. Safety, therefore, addresses processes designed to reduce risk of harm among patients and may be considered the fertile ground from which quality can grow.

Over the years, regulatory and accrediting bodies have become increasingly vigilant in ensuring that hospitals and other healthcare settings comply with accepted safety requirements, particularly around issues of reducing errors. In 2002, TJC established its National Patient Safety Goals (NPSGs) program to help accredited organizations address specific areas of concern in regards to patient safety. Different NPSGs are expected for different practice settings (e.g., hospitals, ambulatory care, behavioral health, long term care) and are considered critical to TJC promotion and enforcement of patient safety standards throughout the health care delivery system (TJC, 2015).

The specific NPSGs are developed with the input of a panel of widely recognized experts called the Patient Safety Advisory Group, composed of nurses, physicians, pharmacists, risk managers, clinical engineers, and other professionals who have hands-on experience in addressing patient safety issues in a wide variety of healthcare settings. Distinct NPSGs are available for hospital, ambulatory, and other settings. TJC routinely reviews, revises, and replaces NPSGs to ensure that they remain current with healthcare practices.

Among the current NPSGs for hospitals is Goal 1: improve the accuracy of patient identification. The rationale for this goal is to reduce chances of wrong-patient errors occurring during diagnosis and treatment. Clearly, this goal addresses one of the fundamental issues raised in the IOM's *To Err is Human* report. Goal 1 is further divided into two specific items: (1) use at least two patient identifiers when providing care, treatment, and service, and (2) eliminate transfusion errors related to patient misidentification. Hospitals are expected to develop procedures and processes that satisfy the objectives of the goal, collect data to demonstrate that they have complied with the goal, and routinely report the data to maintain accreditation by TJC (2015).

Data for Assessing Achievement of Performance and Management/Financial Targets

Hospitals and healthcare organizations have their own internal performance metrics, which include operational data, such as those assessing financial performance, hospital efficiency in terms of throughput, and quality data, such as publicly reported measures recording hospital performance.

Financial data that track hospital inpatient and outpatient volume, number of surgeries, census of inpatient units, and adherence to budgeted targets, are all measures of the profitability of the organization. Hospital profitability is important for nurses to understand, as it is a measure of the financial strength of the organization, and thus an approximate measure of job security.

Operational data that measure hospital efficiency, such as the turnaround time between operative procedures, the time for housekeeping to clean an empty room (and the resultant time to bring a patient from the emergency department to the empty bed), and the number of hospital discharges achieved before noon, all measure the ability of the interconnected systems of care. Operational measures reflect the efficiency of the teams that care for patients: nurses, physicians, and therapists, as well as the support systems such as housekeeping, pharmacy, and food services. The complex systems in hospitals must work together to ensure that patients receive the care they need when they need it.

The quality and performance improvement efforts among interdisciplinary teams in hospitals must measure and track a variety of data in order to improve their standing in these measures. Since the public can now determine the hospital they wish to frequent based on these data, quality management and performance improvement departments focus their attention on collecting and reporting internal data to provide a more real-time view of performance to improve care to patients. Many hospitals have electronic dashboards where organization-specific and unit-specific data can be shared so that staff can follow their progress in improving care to patients. Depending on the philosophical perspective of the management team, data are more or less transparent to others in the hospital.

Data to Support Accreditation: Magnet and The Joint Commission
Magnet Hospital Program

The Magnet hospital program, sponsored by the American Nurses Credentialing Center (ANCC), the certification arm of the ANA, is a strong endorsement of nursing quality and is only issued to the top hospitals in the nation and internationally. Achieving Magnet status is recognition of quality nursing care, as well as teamwork and collaboration among all health professions. The Magnet Recognition Program® advances three goals within healthcare organizations (ANCC, 2015):

1. Promoting quality in a setting that supports professional practice
2. Identifying excellence in the delivery of nursing services to patients/residents
3. Disseminating best practices in nursing services

A Magnet healthcare environment achieves the quality indicators and nursing practice standards outlined in ANA's *Nursing Administration: Scope and Standards of Practice* and other foundational documents (ANA, 2010; McClure, Poulin, Sovie & Wandelt, 1983). The Magnet Recognition Program has five components: (i) Transformational Leadership, (ii) Structural Empowerment, (iii) Exemplary Professional Practice, (iv) New Knowledge, Innovation and Improvements, and (v) Empirical Quality Results (ANCC, 2014). Organizations must meet rigorous requirements for demonstrating quality of care in order to achieve and maintain Magnet status.

Several quality indicators are required for Magnet hospitals. These include policies and procedures (structure and process measures) that describe what nurses do and how they do it; as well as outcome measures, such as what has been achieved. For example, professional certification has been demonstrated to have a positive impact on quality of care (McHugh , Berez, & Small, 2013; Kendall-Gallagher, Aiken, Sloane, & Cimiotti, 2011). An organization may share its policy on certification (structure—how it supports nurses to achieve certification), procedures (process—how nurses obtain certification), and outcomes (what number of certifications have been achieved each year, per unit).

Magnet hospitals address improvements in care, including nurse-sensitive outcomes, such as falls and hospital-acquired pressure ulcers. Magnet hospitals must have programs in place to reduce HACs that demonstrate the role of nurses in driving improvements to care. The evidence base for nurses' role in reducing hospital falls is quite robust (AHRQ, 2013). Falls reduction programs may include risk assessment through instruments such as Morse Falls Scale (Morse, 1989), Hendrich II Fall Risk Model (Hendrich, 2013), and others. The nurse's admission assessment is documented, perhaps in an electronic record, and forms the basis for specific interventions to reduce falls. It is expected that these nursing interventions are implemented 100% of the time, and the effectiveness of these interventions is documented in the medical record. If a patient does fall, an immediate "huddle" should occur with those nurses and ancillary staff present on the shift to determine if there was a deviation from the planned interventions, or if the patient's condition changed and required a different intervention. This qualitative assessment helps to engage all nurses and ancillary staff on the appropriate patient care requirements. This one fall is documented in a database, per the usual event reporting. Any additional falls that day, week, or month are similarly entered into a database. It would then be an expected professional competency for the nurses on that unit to review on a daily, weekly, or monthly basis the number of falls that occurred, possible patient characteristics that may be similar or different, such as age diagnosis, time of day, and number of staff available on the unit. This review is essential in determining what errors were made in the care delivery system to allow the patient to fall, and thus be harmed while under nurses' care. The assessment may not have been accurate or robust enough. The falls prevention intervention may not have been performed correctly. A review of falls data requires more than just numbers. It requires knowledge of the context of the fall, information about the complex factors that may have contributed to the fall, and the wisdom to integrate all of these details in order to come to a conclusion about the effectiveness of the care delivered and formulate an action plan to prevent future falls. This is a simple example of the power of clinical nurses owning their data about their nursing care. Imagine the power of 3 million nurses examining their data on their nursing care delivery each day and using their knowledge and expertise to solve patient problems!

Data to Inform Improvement through Lean Six Sigma

Many hospitals have further developed operational efficiency programs using a Toyota Production program called Lean Six Sigma (Arthur, 2011; Kenney, 2010). This program trains leaders as experts in efficiency and performance improvement, called black belts, who assist their colleagues in identifying inefficiencies in care processes so that patients receive the most streamlined care. Lean suggests the use of care protocols, or best practices, and requires teams to hardwire those practices. Teams perform rapid improvement events to identify the value in the care processes and to eliminate those steps or processes that reflect "the way we have always done it" as opposed to a more innovative best practice. Once the appropriate steps are agreed upon, the team delivers care in the newly-designed process and tracks deviations from the recommended practice. These practice deviations might manifest themselves in putting a piece of equipment in the wrong place or using too many sponges in a dressing. The unit manager plays an important role in ensuring that the new systems are followed and tracks adherence as a measure of unit performance. Lean assumes that all care providers and team members, from nurses and doctors to housekeepers and maintenance engineers, know their role and perform it to the exact specifications outlined, 100% of the time. Deviations are discussed in team rounds to determine if the change in procedure reflects an improvement to the system.

Evidence-based Practice ≠ Quality Data

There is much in the literature and in practice settings on evidence-based practice. Evidence-based practice reflects the synthesis of available research on the topic, with clinical judgment and patient/family preference (AHRQ. Accessed on January 21, 2015. http://effectivehealthcare. ahrq.gov/glossary-of-terms/?pageaction=showterm&termid=24). Linked to requisite improvements in the delivery of health care, evidence-based practice called for providers to harness the available evidence from published studies and implement these findings into practice. Fueled by the seminal IOM work, such as Crossing the Quality Chasm (http://www.nap.edu/books/0309072808/html/), adopting the prevailing evidence cited in published studies, and the resultant protocols, was believed (and still is today) to be an important step to practicing evidence-based health care. The hypothesis is that if one practices according to published evidence, the resultant patient care outcomes will improve. However, in spite of many significant advances, nurses still have more to do to achieve evidence-based practice across the board. A recent survey of the state of evidence-based practice in nurses indicated that, while nurses had positive attitudes toward evidence-based practice and wished to gain more knowledge and skills, they still faced significant barriers in employing it in practice (Melnyk, Fineout-Overholt, Gallagher-Ford, & Kaplan, 2012).

The concept of practice-based evidence provides an interesting alternative to the synthesis of research findings into practice. It assumes the richness of the practice environment to then inform further research. This form of improvement science is another component of practice informing research. Davidoff and Batalden (2005) describe the differences between research and improvement and offer a model to expand the publication of work that is designed to improve the performance of healthcare systems. They note the failure to publish improvement project work results as a serious deficiency in the development of an improvement science, as it limits the available evidence on efficacy, prevents critical scrutiny, deprives staff of the opportunity and incentive to clarify thinking, slows dissemination of established improvements, inhibits discovery of innovations, and compromises the ethical obligation to return valuable information to the public (Davidoff & Batalden, 2005).

Predictive Models in Quality and Safety Improvement
The availability of large databases of patient-level data, collected predominantly through electronic health records and insurance claims data, offers many opportunities to conduct secondary analyses on these valuable data. In addition, there is growing interest in utilizing sophisticated statistical procedures to examine the clinical and statistical significance of trends and correlation among variables that impact quality. Multivariate statistics allow examination of multiple variables together to better understand the influence that one variable has on another or to examine how several variables influence one or more outcome variables. The application of multivariate statistics is multivariate analysis.

Multivariate analyses typically go beyond bivariate analyses, such as crosstabs, which examine the relationship between two variables. Multivariate analysis of variance examines cases where there is more than one dependent variable to be analyzed simultaneously. Multiple regression analyses are used to produce models that try to describe how different variables may impact, or respond simultaneously to, particular outcomes. The multiple regression models can identify the variables that have the greatest impact on desired outcomes and those can be used to predict particular outcomes. These predictive models have great implications in designing improvement projects because they can isolate the characteristics of patients or processes that contribute most significantly to the needed improvement. In many cases, the predictive models indicate which patients are most at risk for particular undesirable outcomes.

Hospital readmission is one of the most important issues in health care, and it has been studied by many (Kansagara et al., 2011). There are several available predictive models that identify the characteristics of patients most likely to be re-hospitalized within 30–60 days.

Acute Care Models to Predict Readmissions

A recent systematic review of the literature on risk prediction models for hospital readmissions conducted by the Health Services Research and Development Service of the Department of Veterans Affairs summarized the types of data being used to develop hospitalization risk models and the available evidence on the effectiveness of the models currently in use (Kansagara et al., 2011). The study examined 26 unique models; 25 of these models focused on 30-day readmission and one was designed to address preventable readmissions. Most of the models relied on *retrospective* administrative data to identify readmission risk. Smaller groups of models were used to predict high-risk patients for intervention during hospitalization or at discharge. Among the common data elements used in these models were: medical comorbidity, prior utilization patterns, and social and demographic factors. The study concluded that despite the variety of predictive models currently in use, there is no clear evidence that they perform well in actually reducing re-hospitalizations and that additional work is needed in this area.

Home Care Models to Predict Readmissions

Preventing hospitalization is one of the major objectives of hospital and home health care (Rosati & Huang, 2007). National estimates indicate

that approximately one-fifth of all home healthcare patients are hospitalized or receive emergent care following admission, though the figure
has been falling since 2007 when it was closer to one-quarter (Gerhardt
et al., 2013). Visiting Nurse Service of New York sought to reduce their
re-hospitalization rates by developing a predictive model that would
allow clinicians to identify patients at risk of hospitalization so that nurses
could intervene appropriately (Russell, Rosenfeld, Ames, & Rosati, 2010).
A team of research staff used patient information from the OASIS, plan
of care, medication review, and medical records to build and validate a
predictive model to estimate a patient's risk of being hospitalized within
60 days following admission to Visiting Nursing Services of New York
(VNSNY). In comparison to hospital risk score, which typically examines 30-day re-admissions, the home care model covers a 60-day time
interval that represents the typical home care episode of care. Analyses
revealed that patients who had a previous history of home health care,
emergent care, or hospitalization and a high number of certified visits
were at significantly higher risk for hospitalization. Clinical factors were
also highly predictive of hospitalization. Among those that significantly
predicted increased risk were unhealed pressure or stasis ulcers, urinary
incontinence, urinary catheters, respiratory symptoms, severe shortness
of breath, and congestive heart failure (Rosati & Huang, 2007). The
predictive model allowed the researchers to categorize patients into seven
risk categories: very low, low, low–moderate, moderate, moderate–high,
high, and very high. The hospitalization risk score made a significant,
improved impact on the quality and clinical practice at VNSNY (Russell
et al., 2010).

Another example of predictive modeling is found in the work of Bekelis,
Bakhoum, Desai, Mackenzie, Goodney, & Labropoulos (2013) who
attempted to develop a risk factor-based predictive model of outcomes
for patients undergoing carotid endarterectomy (CEA). They used data
from 2005–2010 from the American College of Surgeons National
Quality Improvement Project database and found that these patients
demonstrated a 1.64% risk of stroke, 0.69% risk of myocardial infarction, and 0.75% risk of death within 30 days after CEA. Multivariate
analysis demonstrated that a variety of factors contributed to the like-
lihood of negative outcomes including increasing age, sex, history of
chronic obstructive pulmonary disease, myocardial infarction, angina,
congestive heart failure, and others. Additional modeling found a steep
affect of age on the risk of myocardial infarction and death. In short,
the multiple regression analysis helped identify the clinical and personal

characteristics associated with poor outcomes of CEA, such as risk of myocardial infarction and death.

Data Collected for Research Purposes

Typically, the data used for predictive models may be characterized as secondary analysis. There are also primary research studies that collect new data to understand and improve quality nursing care in hospitals. An important example of an organization devoted to conducting scientific research on quality improvement in hospitals is the Improvement Science Research Network (ISRN). The ISRN is the only National Institutes of Health (NIH)-supported improvement research network. The ISRN's primary mission is to accelerate interprofessional improvement science in a systems context across multiple sites. The uniqueness of the ISRN is that its focus on organizational systems makes it possible to scientifically explore the system's effect(s) on the delivery of health care in the acute care setting. The mission of the ISRN is to advance the scientific foundation for quality improvement, safety, and efficiency through trans-disciplinary research addressing healthcare systems, patient-centeredness, and integration of evidence into practice. ISRN studies seek to conduct research on identifying facilitators and barriers to providing quality nursing care in hospitals. The findings of these studies are then used to devise improvement action plans for individual nursing units or entire hospitals and systems.

Recent ISRN studies illustrate how researchers design rigorous studies to learn how to understand and improve quality of nursing processes in hospitals. One study, "Small Troubles, Adaptive Responses (STAR-2): Frontline Nurse Engagement in Quality Improvement," explores the types and frequency of first order operational failures that nurses self-detect during their work shifts. Nurses on participating units at partnering hospitals collect data in real time on small operational failures and then solve these problems to deliver safe care.

Another ISRN study, "Team Performance for Patient Safety" (TeamSTEPPS), is an evidence-based system aimed at improving patient outcomes by fostering improvements in teamwork and communication skills among members of the healthcare team. This study focused on the effectiveness of TeamSTEPPS as an improvement science demonstration model and examined the dynamics of teams working in real-world clinical settings. The approach was found to be helpful in identifying gaps in knowledge and practice with regard to optimal teamwork.

In conclusion, there are many types of data collection activities that nurses, government, and other stakeholders examine to assess the quality and safety of nursing care. This data has many functions, including compliance and regulatory requirements; assuring standardized care, that can be compared across units and institutions; developing predictive risk models; and improving the science of quality nursing care. These efforts offer a rich collection of information from primary and secondary sources and create an infinite number of analyses and interpretations for institution-wide improvement effort.

Quality and Safety Data in Home Health Care

Hospitals have been the primary focus of research and literature of quality and safety in health care. There are many commonalities across healthcare settings about quality and safety, as well as the measurement of desired patient outcomes. However, it is important to emphasize that the goals of home health services are different from those of acute care settings. Home care aims to help individuals live with greater independence and assist the patient with avoiding hospitalization or admission to long-term care institutions. Moreover, some home healthcare patients are on a trajectory of decline and possess a decreased ability to carry out activities of daily living (ADLs), so "an implicit goal of home health care is to facilitate a supported decline" (Ellenbecker, Samia, Cushman, & Alster, 2008).

Health care in the home is predominantly delivered by nurses with less physician contact than in hospitals. Typically, physicians rely on nurses to make assessments and communicate findings. In addition, because the care takes place in the patient's home, respect for patient autonomy is an important consideration, and home healthcare patients and their caregivers are often more engaged in determining what the goals of their care should be. In comparison to hospitals, where nurses are consistently in contact with patients and can monitor care regimens and quality and safety practices, home health nurses are not in a position to monitor patient behavior when they leave the home. Thus, the patient may choose to adopt practices that result in poor outcomes, or which may be contrary to best practices. Similarly, many home care patients receive care from family members and other informal caregivers who may not fully understand the importance of adhering to quality and safety standards. In short, home health nurses confront many challenges in maintaining quality and safety standards in delivering care in the privacy of a patient's home (Ellenbecker et al., 2008).

"Medicare-certified" means the home health agency is approved by Medicare and meets certain federal health and safety requirements. Beginning in 2000, Medicare-certified home health agencies use a standardized assessment tool at the start and end of each care episode called OASIS (Outcome-Assessment and Information Set) and OBQI (outcome-based quality improvement) to track and monitor quality. This standardized approach to data collection allows providers to monitor, report, and benchmark quality and safety measures such as falls, pressure ulcers, and declines in functional status. Evidence is growing to support interventions to improve quality for home health care in several key areas. Below is a brief description of five quality and safety indicators most relevant to home care and some of the current approaches for addressing improvements (Ellenbecker et al., 2008; Rosati, 2009):

1. Medication management and prevention of medication errors/ adverse effect of poly-pharmacy: RNs perform medication reconciliation for patients with five or more medications; telephone or video reminders have been found useful.

2. Fall prevention: Importance of risk assessment, physical therapy to improve gait and balance; recognize that falls may be the result of specific drugs.

3. Unplanned hospital admissions: A primary goal of home health care is to avoid subsequent hospitalizations; yet, despite many descriptive studies, there are few evidence-based practices to reduce unplanned readmissions.

4. Functional status: Maintaining or improving functional status is a key outcome measure in home care, and descriptive studies suggest that working closely with and supporting family caregivers can impact functional status and help patients remain in their homes. Research studies have also indicated that use of technology and electronic communication, as well as working with APN colleagues, can be effective in delaying or reducing admissions to long-term care facilities.

5. Wound and pressure ulcer management: Over one-third of home health patients are treated for pressure ulcers. Assessment and treatment of wounds, as well as prevention of new wounds, reflect an important quality indicator of home health care.

Clearly, nurse-sensitive indicators in home care overlap with hospital-focused indicators. Failure to meet quality standards related to falls, wound care, and other aspects of home care can result in hospitalizations.

However, though similarities exist, there are unique features in home care that make it difficult to simply transfer research findings from one setting to the next. Because of these variations, home care providers must advance their own quality and safety initiatives, as well as define their own measures for monitoring and assessing their outcomes specific to their practices.

As mentioned, Home Health Compare is similar to Hospital Compare in that it has information about the quality of care provided by Medicare-certified home health agencies throughout the nation. Home Health Compare can help patients and their family or friends choose a quality home health agency that has the skilled home health services needed, and home health agencies and healthcare professionals can use Home Health Compare (see Sidebar 2.2) to do the following:

- Review the performance of agencies in a particular area
- Identify opportunities for quality improvement
- Answer patients' questions and educate them about their choices

There are three types of Home Health Quality Measures, which are roughly based on the Donebedian model:

1. Process Measures
2. Outcome Measures
3. Potentially Avoidable Events

These measures are designed to reflect distinctive home care nursing practices. Process measures have been publicly reported since October 2010 and Outcome and Potentially Avoidable Event measures have been reported since June 2011. Beginning in January 2014, claims-based measures of rehospitalization and emergency department use without hospital readmission during the first 30 days of home health will be included in publicly reported outcome measures (see Sidebar 2.2).

Who Decides What Constitutes Quality and How to Measure It?
In the aftermath of the IOM studies, there has been significant progress in identifying quality indicators associated with nursing practice (Savitz, Jones, & Bernard, 2005). Research on the relationship between the nursing workforce and workplace conditions on quality outcomes provides compelling evidence that particular patient outcomes are directly

SIDEBAR 2.2

HOME HEALTH COMPARE

Selected Measures

Process Measures	As listed on Home Health Compare
Timely initiation of care	How often the home health team began their patients' care in a timely manner.
Influenza immunization received for current flu season	How often the home health team determined whether patients received a flu shot for the current flu season.
Pneumococcal polysaccharide vaccine ever received	How often the home health team determined whether their patients received a pneumococcal vaccine (pneumonia shot).
Heart failure symptoms addressed	How often the home health team treated heart failure (weakening of the heart) patients' symptoms.
Diabetic foot care and patient education implemented	For patients with diabetes, how often the home health team got doctor's orders, gave foot care, and taught patients about foot care.
Pain assessment conducted	How often the home health team checked patients for pain.
Pain interventions implemented	How often the home health team treated their patients' pain.
Depression assessment conducted	How often the home health team checked patients for depression.
Drug education on all medications provided to patient/caregiver	How often the home health team taught patients (or their family caregivers) about their drugs.
Multifactor fall risk assessment conducted for all patients who can ambulate	How often the home health team checked patients' risk of falling.
Pressure ulcer risk conducted	How often the home health team checked patients for the risk of developing pressure sores (bed sores).
Pressure ulcer prevention included in the plan of care	How often the home health team included treatments to prevent pressure sores (bed sores) in the plan of care.
Pressure ulcer prevention implemented	How often the home health team took doctor-ordered action to prevent pressure sores (bed sores).

HOME HEALTH COMPARE (CONT'D)

Outcome Measures

Outcome Measures	As listed on Home Health Compare
Improvement in ambulation	How often patients got better at walking or moving around
Improvement in bed transfer	How often patients got better at getting in and out of bed
Improvement in pain interfering with activity	How often patients had less pain when moving around
Improvement in bathing	How often patients got better at bathing
Improvement in management of oral medications	How often patients got better at taking their drugs correctly by mouth
Improvement in dyspnea	How often patients' breathing improved
Improvement in status of surgical wounds	How often patients' wounds improved or healed after an operation
Acute care hospitalizations	How often home health patients had to be admitted to the hospital
Emergency department use without hospitalization	How often patients receiving home health care needed any urgent, unplanned care in the hospital emergency room—without being admitted to the hospital

Source: Center for Medicare & Medicaid Services (CMS). List of quality measures (http://www.medicare.gov/HomeHealthCompare/Data/Quality-Measures-List.html)

related to adequacy of nursing staff (Clarke & Aiken, 2003; Kovner & Gergen, 1998; Needleman et al., 2011). The term nursing-sensitive indicators (Maas, Johnson, & Moorhead, 1996) identified those negative or adverse outcomes associated with nursing care, including medication errors, patient falls, and nosocomial infections. The term nurse-sensitive indicators, which has broad implications, has been adopted widely, though its focus is predominantly on a nurse's ability to reduce harm and negative outcomes (Haberfelde, Bedecarre & Buffum (2005) . Research that examines the positive outcomes associated with nursing care is far less common (Needleman et al., 2011).

Federal Agencies and Non-Governmental Organizations Agencies
AHRQ

The Agency for Healthcare Research and Quality (AHRQ), a government agency housed in the U.S., Department of Health and Human Services (DHHS) has devoted many resources to understanding, measuring, and researching quality in health care. AHRQ adopted a wide and varied approach for identifying indicators of quality, which required multiple cycles of comprehensive reviews of the literature; extensive data mining of government databases, such as Healthcare Cost and Utilization Project (HCUP); analysis of claims data for specific ICD-9 diagnostic grouping; and integration of input from a wide range of academic, research, and clinical experts across the healthcare spectrum (see Figure 1).

AHQR has developed the most comprehensive package of quality indicators (QIs). The QIs are evidence-based measures of quality of care provided on an inpatient and outpatient basis. The measures are organized into four modules: Prevention Quality Indicators (PQIs), Inpatient Quality Indicators (IQIs), Patient Safety Indicators (PSIs), and Pediatric Quality Indicators (PDIs) (AHRQ, 2015). Current uses of the AHRQ quality indicators include: (i) using comparative data to measure performance of different hospitals on specific measures, (ii) identification of quality improvement initiatives within healthcare settings, (iii) public reporting purposes, such as pay for performance (P4P), and (iv) research.

As outlined on their website, the AHRQ data have relevance to nurses because of their focus on measuring both past and current performance to help guide future improvement projects. Current demands for quality tracking, measurement, reporting, and linking payment to quality are the result of efforts of governments, accrediting bodies, purchasers, and others to effect change. Nurses are not only members of the quality team, but they also often lead and coordinate conceptualization and imple-ment quality and improvement initiatives. Nurses are well positioned to review and interpret performance data as well as design interventions to improve quality of care (Farquhar, 2008).

To be sure, data availability is an issue that plagues many hospitals and other healthcare settings. Typical data sources include clinical data, administrative data, survey data, and operational data, each with its

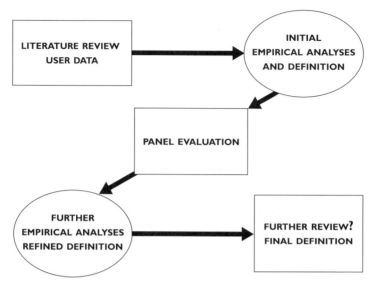

FIGURE 1. The AHRQ Quality Indicator Development and Evaluation Process
(*Source:* Farquhar, 2008)

own strengths and limitations. Administrative data are the most widely available source of information about hospital services, patient care, and patient outcomes, since all hospitals generate such data as part of billing operations. However, as AHRQ officials acknowledge, the data lacks the depth of clinical detail that can help measure quality, and variations in coding practices may create challenges for quality evaluation.

Nurses need to be clear about their objectives in using AHRQ or other quality measures: is it for quality improvement or public accountability? Or pay for performance (P4P)? Each audience and stakeholder group may have somewhat different interests or uses for quality data. Nurses can serve an important role in designing measurement strategies and/or quality improvement programs. Additionally, nurses are well positioned to analyze data from measures and design and implement strategies that impact care delivery.

National Quality Forum

The National Quality Forum (NQF) is a nonprofit, "membership-based organization that works to catalyze improvements in health care," (NQF, 2015). NQF endorsements signify top quality evidence-based health care and help improve patient safety and maternity care, achieve better outcomes, strengthen chronic care management, and keep healthcare costs down. A membership-based forum, NQF includes a wide array of consumers, purchasers, professionals, providers, and other organizations, such as labor unions, accrediting bodies, research organizations, and supporting industries. The NQF has focused on several areas of healthcare improvement, specifically error rates, unnecessary procedures, and under-treatment, especially regarding preventative care. The NQF has defined six types of "never events" or Serious Reportable Events and recommends a national reporting system for such events in order to improve patient care quality.

The six types of "never events" (officially called Serious Reportable Events) are:

1. Surgical events (e.g., surgery performed on the wrong patient),
2. Product or device events (e.g., using contaminated drugs),
3. Patient protection events (e.g., an infant discharged to the wrong person),
4. Care management events (e.g., a medication error),
5. Environmental events (e.g., electric shock or burn), and
6. Criminal events (e.g., sexual assault of a patient).

Monitoring of these never events has been integrated into quality programs in most hospitals and, when applicable, other healthcare delivery settings.

National Database for Nursing Quality Indicators

The National Database for Nursing Quality Indicators (NDNQI) is the only national nursing quality measurement program that enables you to compare measures of your nursing quality against national, regional, and state norms for hospitals of your type down to the unit level (see Sidebar 2.3). Used by more than 2,000 hospitals nationwide, it is the largest provider of unit-level performance data to hospitals. NDNQI data allows staff nurses and nursing leadership the chance to review their data and evaluate nursing performance relative to patient outcomes. Your facility can use the information to establish organizational goals for improvement at the unit level. Comparisons exist for Magnet®/Non-Magnet, Case Mix Index, and many others. You can mark your progress in improving the care of patients and the work environment of nurses, avoid costly complications, and help market the quality of your care.

SIDEBAR 2.3

NDNQI QUALITY MEASURES

Enabling Unit-level Quality Comparisons

NDNQI's quality measures reported at the unit level include: fall/injury fall rates; hospital-/unit-acquired pressure ulcer rates; nursing hours per patient day; nursing skill mix; physical restraint prevalence; peripheral IV infiltration rate; RN education/certification; assault/injury assault rates; pain assessment/intervention/reassessment cycles completed; ventilato r-associated pneumonia rate; central line–associated bloodstream infection rate; catheter-associated urinary tract infection rate; nurse turnover rate.

New Clinical Measures in 2014

- Falls in ambulatory settings (now available)

- Pressure ulcer incidence rates from electronic health records (now available)

- Nursing care hours in emergency departments, Perioperative Units and perinatal units

- Hospital readmission rates

- Skill mix in emergency departments, Perioperative units and Perinatal units

Source: Press Ganey (n.d.) (http://www.nursingquality.org/About-NDNQI/ Quality-Data-Solutions)

Registered Nurse Satisfaction

RN satisfaction is another metric reported by the NDNQI and benchmarked against the national database. The same benchmarks of Magnet/ non-Magnet organizations, as well as hospital bed size are available for reporting. These benchmarks help nurses and leadership understand performance against a national norm. How satisfied nurses are with their practice environment and their work environment are important indicators for a safety culture. Nurses, as the largest healthcare workforce, have the most influence on quality and safety for hospitals. If nurses rate their satisfaction lower than other hospitals, the research suggests that the hospital will have worse patient outcomes than hospitals with nurses who are highly satisfied (Aiken, 2011). Hospital leaders who do not address low RN satisfaction are at great risk for losing patients, doctors, nurses, and market-share. Quality, including RN satisfaction, is just good business.

NDNQI offers four RN survey options:

- RN Survey with Practice Environment Scale
- RN Survey with Job Satisfaction Scales – R
- RN Survey with Job Satisfaction Scales
- RN Survey with Job Satisfaction Scales – Short Form

The measures of Nursing Hours per Patient Day (NHPPD), skill mix, falls, and falls with injury were submitted by ANA to NQF and are part of the NQF-endorsed nursing-sensitive care measure set. ANA is the measure steward for these four measures, and this guideline provides the micro-specifications for those measures. The ANA measures were re-endorsed by the NQF in August 2009 and May 2012. This is a strong example of how nursing influences both the quality and policy agendas and demonstrates acceptance of the data that links nurses to quality of care.

There are many organizations and associations dedicated to identifying and examining quality measures in health care. Moreover, there seems to be consensus about the nursing practices and work processes that are associated with positive patient outcomes. Nonetheless, there is little evidence of consistency in how nurse-sensitive outcomes are defined and measured across different groups using different tools and data elements. Savitz and colleagues (2005) conducted a systematic review of quality indicators sensitive to nurse staffing in acute care and found:

- Lack of standardized performance measure definition
- Lack of consensus on a core set of evidence-based measurements
- Limited availability of data at the unit and/or shift level

Among their recommendations is a call to look beyond nurse staffing as the primary structural measure for quality care and focus on positive outcomes associated with nursing care. This is opposed to the current emphasis, which focuses exclusively on monitoring nurses' contributions to reducing harm from events such as falls, medication errors, hospital-acquired infections, and pressure ulcers.

Conclusion

Measuring quality is a complex process that requires a consensus-driven, clear, standardized definition of data elements associated with nursing processes and outcomes. Many public and private organizations are devoted to identifying appropriate indicators to measure quality processes and outcomes in health care. Understanding the methods of collecting and interpreting quality data is critical to achieving desired outcomes. Nurse-sensitive indicators are specific patient outcomes associated with nursing practice and include falls, pressure ulcers, hospital-acquired infections, and restraint use. These indicators are a subset of a long and varied list of processes and outcome measures in health care. Though differences exist in nursing standards of care across hospitals, home care agencies, skilled nursing homes, and community settings, there are shared measures and shared expectations across the healthcare spectrum.

3

Utilizing Data to Inform Patient Care and Track Outcomes: Answering the Question, *How Are We Doing?*

Most nurses have had some experience collecting or reviewing data on quality and safety at their institutions. Obtaining data for public reporting and other purposes is often considered a critical part of the nursing role. Measures, especially those characterized as nurse-sensitive indicators, are deeply rooted in nursing practices in all healthcare settings, and many organizations have Nurse Quality Departments or groups devoted to monitoring and reporting data and trends. However, these data alone do not provide a complete answer to "How are we doing?" When one institution's data is compared to another's, it is possible to determine how well each one is doing relative to the other. When many comparable institutions collect and report the same data, it is possible to better interpret and understand the performance of each institution.

A simple illustration of these sorts of comparisons is the Hospital Compare website, as described in Chapter 2 (also Home Health Compare and Physician Compare). These websites provide graphics and figures that depict how several institutions compare on specific quality indicators, so that consumers can easily observe which hospital has the best scores. In other words, these data represent performance of the different institutions. However, being "better" than one or two selected hospitals does not necessarily translate into higher-quality care. Hospital Compare allows consumers to explore how one hospital compares to other hospitals in the same city or state, which offers the ability to understand how one hospital measures up to hospitals in larger geographic areas. These kinds of comparisons have limited utility in assessing quality, which should be determined by comparing individual performance to best practices, benchmarks, or targets that would provide a more complete answer as to how well the institution is measuring up to professional or regulatory standards. This chapter will explore the relevance of these approaches and their implications to nursing practice.

First, a note about *units of analysis*. The unit of analysis is the "who" or the "what" that you are analyzing or studying. Often the unit of analysis is the patient, but it is not unusual for data to be collected on specific providers (RNs, MDs, pharmacists, etc.) or types of institutions (hospitals, home care, and skilled nursing facilities). When one is measuring quality, it is critical that you compare data using the same unit of analysis: patients to patients, nurses to nurses, etc.

Moreover, it is important that the units of analysis are as closely alike as possible so that the comparisons are meaningful. For example, most healthcare institutions collect data on how many patients had hospital-acquired pressure ulcers (HAPU). This number could be reported as a total for the entire hospital, by individual units within the hospital, or by types of patient (e.g., medical vs. surgical). But, it is not appropriate to compare HAPU in an academic medical center to, say, HAPU in a psychiatric hospital since the two institutions are not comparable with respect to likelihoods of developing HAPU. Similarly, it might not make as much sense to compare HAPU in children to HAPU in adults in the ICU. For these reasons quality data, such as NDNQI, is typically reported by groupings that have something in common: surgical units are compared to other surgical units, ICUs to ICUs, and so on.

Learning from Other Industries

As quality and safety concerns became increasingly important in health care, it became apparent that other industries had already made significant strides in understanding how to study and reduce risks of negative outcomes. The aviation industry provided an excellent starting point to better understand how to reduce errors and risks. Lessons learned from aviation echoed some of the conclusions of the IOM reports and also offered insights on integrating safety principles into day-to-day operations in complex organizations, such as hospitals. Some of the critical safety principles learned from aviation include:

1. Errors typically occur from faulty systems, not individual negligence;
2. Accident prevention must be ongoing and based on open reporting, that is, blameless and transparent reporting of adverse events; and
3. Major accidents might be rare but near misses and other incidents, which are less apparent, can signal deeper problems in the organization (Wilf-Miron, Lewenhoff, Benyamini, & Aviram, 2003; DeKorne, vanWijngaarden, Hiddema, Bleeker, Pronovost & Klanzinga, 2010).

These principles form the foundation for many nursing quality initiatives. However, progress on improving quality and safety in health care has not been as sustained and effective as it has been in aviation, where all stakeholders have embraced common practices to reduce the likelihoods of crashes and other aviation crises. Pronovost and colleagues (2009) suggest several reasons for the sluggish progress in reducing harm and increasing quality in health care as compared to innovations in aviation. Firstly, an error in health care results in negative outcomes for individual patients; when an error occurs in aviation, hundreds of fatalities may result. In addition, efforts to implement risk reduction practices in aviation are typically restricted to a limited number of individuals (mechanics, pilots) in particular locations (cockpits, engines) and times (landing and takeoff); in health care, the risk of harm or error can be found in many areas and among different providers. Another reason for the slow pace of change in health care may be due to the varying levels of commitments among healthcare institutions to investing the financial and other resources necessary to study and improve quality and safety. Some of this will change as insurers and payers (such as Medicare and Medicaid) require minimum standards of quality reporting to receive full reimbursement for services.

Lessons have also been learned from retail, sports, banking, and politics, particularly in ways to use data to measure performance and improve quality (McNeill, 2013). For example, nursing's knowledge and appreciation of patient satisfaction has been largely influenced by research among businesses seeking to satisfy customers and attain customer loyalty. Statistics and data are integral parts of sports and demand for empirical evidence of player performance has had some influence on healthcare quality data and analytics, as well. And, in the world of politics, models that predict voter preferences and outcomes have been useful in the development of predictive models to measure risk for many healthcare outcomes. In short, nurses and others in health care have borrowed much from professionals in other industries with regard to applying innovative uses of data for quality and safety purposes.

Dashboards, Scorecards, Targets and Benchmarks

Though nursing and healthcare organizations have adopted a variety of ideas from different industries about using data to measure performance, it is not possible to simply cut and paste from one industry to another. It is critical that performance and outcome measures are examined to provide meaningful information to providers, which typically means that comparisons are examined among similar or like groupings—comparing apples to apples. Different approaches to reporting standardized measures of performance are commonly used in healthcare organizations with the explicit goal of using comparative data to determine "How are we doing?" As described in Chapter 2, there are many public reporting sites designed to allow users to compare performance data across health organizations.

There are many tools that are currently used within organizations to allow individual work units to monitor and assess their performance on quality and safety indicators. Dashboards, scorecards, targets, and benchmarks are increasingly common in nursing and other fields to allow clinicians, managers, and administrators to assess performance on priority indicators and determine where their strengths and weaknesses lie. The data on these tools are vital to the selection of quality improvement projects specific to individual units or services. To be sure, there is some overlap among these different terms, and often they are used interchangeably. Nonetheless, it's helpful to recognize the unique features of each.

Dashboards

Dashboards, as the word suggests, is a term borrowed from the automotive industry. Dashboards are meant to provide at a glance data in key areas, as a driver might quickly look at their dashboard to determine speed, amount of gas, how many miles driven, etc. The key performance indicators (KPI) on the dashboards reflect the particular objectives or business processes being monitored by the individual or institution. Different individuals within an organization are likely to have different dashboards that are unique to their specific responsibilities or their location in the organizational hierarchy. Thus, a nurse manager's dashboard would be different than the dashboard of the Chief Nursing Officer or the

Chief Executive Officer. In addition, it is possible and likely that certain individuals would have many dashboards in order to monitor a wide range of processes (Byrnes, 2012: Spetz, Chu, Lin, Fishman, & Melichar, 2013). For example, the Chief Nursing Officer may examine a dashboard on the progress each unit is making on a discharge before noon initiative and also monitor another that illustrates the current wait time in the ER and in ambulatory settings.

In short, dashboards provide signs that let the user clearly see when something is wrong or something is right. By design, dashboards are typically limited to show summaries, key trends, comparisons, and exceptions. They are often one page (or one screen on the computer) with graphic presentation of current and historical trends on KPI. There are four key elements to a good dashboard:

1. Simple and communicates easily
2. Minimum distractions
3. Supports work processes with meaningful and useful data
4. Applies human visual perception to visual presentation of information

Figures 2 through 4 are examples of one institution's dashboards.

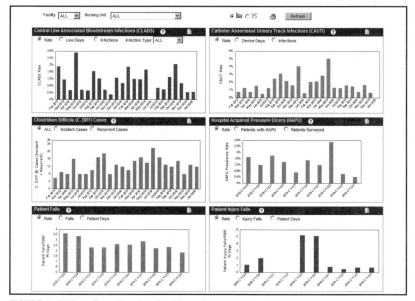

FIGURE 2. Patient Care–Nursing Dashboard

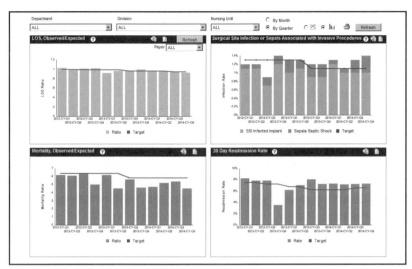

FIGURE 3. Patient Care–Quality Dashboard

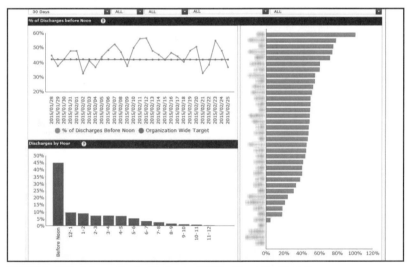

FIGURE 4. Patient Care–Timely Discharge (30-Day View) Dashboard

Scorecards

As the name suggests, scorecards let managers and administrators track the execution of activities of their staff members and monitor the consequences of these actions. Also known as a *balanced scorecard* (BSC), scorecards are used to help managers assess whether their staff is performing within the standards of care defined by the organization

(Hall et al., 2003). Scorecards focus on metrics that reflect the strategic agenda of the organization; identification of a limited number of data elements to monitor a mixture of clinical, financial, and non-financial data elements.

Many healthcare institutions have adopted the use of quality scorecards (see Table 3.1) to measure organizational performance (Kaplan & Norton, 1996). In many cases, scorecards are developed and designed to promote consensus about the desired performance metrics for the organization. Scorecard measures are subject to change as organizational priorities evolve. Indeed, organizations use scorecards explicitly to address areas for improvement and often estimated timelines are included, as well.

Once the metrics are established by leadership or through consensus, providers and clinicians are made aware of the expectations and processes being measured. Typically, some milestone (or target) is established to clearly express the desired level of performance, so that providers and managers can assess how their performance aligns with organizational goals (Kaplan & Norton, 1996).

As illustrated in Table 3.1, the Quality Scorecard developed by Visiting Nurses Service of New York provides a good illustration (Rosati, 2009; Russell et al., 2010) of one that is organized in four categories of clinical performance, including:

1. **Process measures** (e.g., documentation of clinical protocols)
2. **Outcome measures** (e.g., hospitalization rate, wound improvement or deterioration)
3. **Cost measures** (e.g., visits per episode of care)
4. **Patient satisfaction** (e.g., patient–provider communication, overall satisfaction)

The scorecard is populated with data from several sources, including the OASIS and VNSNY information systems, EHRs, payment systems, and a survey on patient satisfaction conducted by an external organization.

VNSNY establishes expected performance levels (targets), and a coding system of colors is used to indicate performance levels on various quality indicators: red symbolizes more than 10% from the target in a negative direction, yellow represents between 10% and the target, and green displays performance at the target or better. With this "traffic light" color

Quality Scorecard

Report Coverage: Jan 2008 to Dec 2008
Program Selected: ALL - All Program (A,C,F,I,L,S)
Region Selected: ALL - All Borough
Team Selected: ALL - All Team

Process Measures	Target	Monthly	Actual YTD
Care Management Documentation (**)	85.0%	86.4%	85.4%
Diabetic Care		87.8%	88.2%
Wound Care		87.9%	85.0%
CHF Care		78.4%	76.9%
HHA Oversight	85.0%	90.0%	87.7%
Supervision is documented every 14 days		90.1%	87.7%
Compliance with completion of HHA Task tool at SOC and Re-evaluation		88.3%	87.9%
Discharge Planning			
Documentation of Discharge plan for patients by 120 days	85.0%	89.4%	92.1%
Submission of Schedule			
% of staff submitting visit schedule timely ++	90.0%	NA	0.0%

Outcomes Measures	Target	Monthly	Actual YTD
All Dx: Overall Hospitalization Rate (**)	28.6%	29.8%	28.6%
% days to hospitalization from SOC/ROC: 1-3 days		6.3%	7.6%
% days to hospitalization from SOC/ROC: 4-30 days		54.9%	52.2%
% days to hospitalization from SOC/ROC: 31-60 days		15.5%	16.8%
% days to hospitalization from SOC/ROC: 61-120 days		9.9%	9.8%
% days to hospitalization from SOC/ROC: >120 days		13.4%	13.6%
All Dx: Overall Hospitalization Rate (Active Census)	8.8%	8.2%	9.1%
Wounds			
Emergent care for wound infections, deteriorating wound status	1.0%	1.2%	1.0%

FIGURE 5. Quality Scorecaard Example (*Source*: Russell, Rosenfeld, Ames, & Rosati, 2010)

scheme, clinicians and managers can instantly see which area represents strength (green) and those areas that require improvement (red).

Targets and Benchmarks

The VNSNY Scorecard includes agency-driven performance expectations or targets for many of their measures. These targets are developed by the leadership to clearly articulate their goals for a given timeframe. In other words, the targets are internally defined by organizational goals that *do not necessarily* reflect external standards set by regulatory agencies or professional associations.

Targets that are set by comparing one organization's processes and performance measures to exemplars or best practices in the industry are known as *benchmarks*. Measures of quality, time, and cost are among the most frequent quality indicators in health care. The process of setting practice benchmarks may involve the identification of industry-wide, consensus-driven indicators, such as nurse-sensitive indicators, that allow one institution to compare their performance processes and outcomes to a larger group of similar organizations. Alternatively, best practice benchmarking involves identification of organizations that are known for exemplary processes and outcomes so that individual organizations may measure their performance as compared to these exemplars. In these ways, institutions can determine how closely they align (or don't align) with industry benchmarks or exemplars.

Clinical Decision Support Systems

As patient-level data becomes increasingly accessible for manifold mandatory reporting and quality performance and improvement, it becomes possible to build clinical decision support for clinicians to use in patient care. Clinical decision support systems (CDSS) are computer programs designed to assist clinicians at the point of care. These systems are designed to be a direct aid to clinical decision-making, in which the characteristics of an individual patient are matched to a computerized clinical knowledge base, and patient-specific assessments or recommendations are then presented to the clinician or the patient for a decision (Mick, 2011). CDSS has been instrumental in a wide range of areas, such as identifying potentially dangerous drug interactions within a patient's medication list.

Clinical decision support systems offer a wider range of options to further enhance patient care. One of the most common is the use of alerts, which notify the clinician of a patient's condition or characteristic that might put them at potential risk. Some examples of alerts include identification of patients at risk of falling or taking medications that are associated with delirium, to name a few.

Some CDSS have evidence-adaptive functions which integrate up-to-date evidence from the research literature and practice-based sources to the point-of care (Sim et al., 2001). For example, a CDSS for cancer treatment is evidence-adaptive if it provides clinicians with information on current evidence and up-to-date practice recommendations for care based on research findings (Sim et al., 2001).

Thus, with the availability of predictive models, institutions can build evidence-adaptive alerts for patients at risk of being re-admitted to the hospital and, once identified, provide evidence-based interventions to prevent the possibility of a negative outcome. The VNSNY predictive hospitalization risk score described in Chapter 2 was integrated into the clinical decision support system at the agency. Each day clinicians received an alert identifying those newly-admitted patients with high hospital readmission risk scores, and specific evidence-based interventions were recommended, such as front-loading visits during the first few weeks of care, ordering remote physiological monitors, and seeking the assistance of an Advanced Practice Nurse. The use of the alerts and the evidence-based clinical support system was found to have an effective, beneficial impact on patient care (Russell et al., 2010).

Relevance for Clinical Nurses and Leaders

The impact of nursing will be realized as nurses gain more knowledge and skill in the use and interpretation of data about their patients, and the care they provide. Data are combined and presented in different groupings for different types of dashboard and report card users. The most specific category for a dashboard would help an individual RN address the clinical status of a patients. One of the widest categories would be dashboard that compares measures across institutions in different geographic areas. A brief description of the types of groupings follows.

Patient Level Data for Use by Registered Nurses

Data are a collection of facts and statistics, collected together for the purpose of analysis. "Data" are plural; a "datum" is the singular form of "data". Data can be considered in a hierarchy: data, information, knowledge, and wisdom (ANA, 2008). Data alone are meaningless; they have to be interpreted, and only then can they be considered information. Knowledge, the next level up, is data that has been interpreted and thus can be synthesized into relationships. The numbers for vital signs: 125/60; heart rate of 70, with respirations of 20, are a set of data. Until we look at the context of these data as an adult or a newborn, with the specific characteristics of the person the data reflect, they are meaningless. But as the vital signs on your patient, reviewed with the prior set of vital signs taken on the previous shift, they provide information that lets you determine if these vital signs are similar to the prior shift or markedly different. Adding a level of relationship to the vital signs, such as temperature, and age, has moved us into the level of knowledge where one may note the patient's history and additional data to determine that the patient may be developing an infection. Finally, wisdom is the appropriate use of knowledge to solve human problems. In the example of vital signs above, the nurse uses their practice experience and expertise to develop a plan for care that addresses the patient's unique individual characteristics.

Unit Level Data for Use by Managers and Directors

Nurses use data every day in their practice, caring for a patient or a group of patients. Nurses need to understand many types of complex data: blood pressure and heart rate, respirations, temperature, intake, and output, all numbers that mean something to the nurse providing care. Nurses juggle numerous points of data on a group of patients: whose blood pressure is up, whose is down. Because our patients are unique individuals, we hold their data separate. However, as nurses we are accountable for the care we deliver, and thus we must look beyond our assigned patients to a group of patients: our unit, our service, our hospital or clinic. These are the data that we as nurses are being held accountable for and what our units, hospitals, clinics, and practices are being measured for. ANA's Social Policy Statement (ANA, 2012) affirms that we serve the public. Our responsibility to the public is that we deliver care that is expert and excellent, and serves to promote both health and healing. Publicly reported data about hospitals is just that—data. Nurses and the public need to be well-versed in interpreting those data, bringing it to the levels of information and knowledge. The care we provide is measurable, and thus the effects of our care can be measured. We as nurses need to be as knowledgeable as our public in order to explain our outcomes.

A representative unit report card is included in Appendix A on page 87.

Institutional Level Data for Leadership

Many measurements of health are publicly available at the local, state, regional, and national levels. Hospitalcompare.gov is a national site where hospital-level data can be compared by patients. Hospital Compare, the CMS website, contains quality data on more than 4,000 hospitals in the United States and is designed for consumers to compare hospitals' quality outcomes on patient experience, timeliness of care, readmissions, complications, and deaths (hospitalcompare.gov). This public reporting of hospital quality data is directly impacted by nursing care and contains metrics that most hospitals track on a monthly or quarterly basis. If your process and outcome measures are available for patients to review, nurses too can review these data. Suggestion: Go to hospitalcompare.gov and find your own hospital, then select a neighboring hospital and see how your hospital compares to your competitor.

Leaders are not only interested in the relative performance of the different units or divisions within their institution. They are also interested in the performance of their institution vis a vis other like-institutions. To properly place an institutions performance among similar institutions, it is useful to use "benchmarks". Benchmarks are aggregated data from many organizations that allow comparisons in cost and other measures across like-institutions. In other words, benchmarks allow specific types of organizations (such as academic medical centers, pediatric hospitals, or magnet designated hospitals) to compare themselves to other organizations with similar characteristics (Sloane Donaldson et al., 2008).

Data on Geographic Regions for Leadership and Policy-Makers

Some states publicly report data. This provides consumers with more local data about care in those hospitals. Several states (NY, CA, TX) now report risk-adjusted outcomes data on a variety of cardiac conditions (Chen, Orav, & Epstein, 2012). New York was one of the first states to publicly report patient outcomes (mortality, etc.) on cardiac surgery. The numbers of cases performed, along with complications and death were reported in the New York Times, causing much anxiety among surgeons, hospitals, and patients for several years (Altman, 1990; Burack, Impellizzeri, Homel, & Cunningham, 1999; Hannan, Stone, Biddle, & DeBuono, 1997). Recent reporting of sepsis and infection rates often linked to low hand hygiene rates, further complicate the landscape for health providers. Several states report data about nurse staffing, either as hours of care provided on an annualized basis (Massachusetts: http://

www.patientcarelink.org/), or some other form of public reporting, internal committees to review nurse staffing which include input from clinical nurses (American Nurses Association, http://www.nursingworld. org/MainMenuCategories/Policy-Advocacy/State/Legislative-Agenda-Reports/State-StaffingPlansRatios). Some cities report hospital data, communicable disease rates, such as influenza, infection rates, and recently, breastfeeding rates (New York City: http://www.nyc.gov/html/ doh/downloads/pdf/ms/breastfeeding-rates-report.pdf).

Data to Inform Policy (ANA)
Finally, data has significant relevance for clinical nurses and leaders in the areas of research, administration, and policy. Here is where data can be the most powerful. Clinical nurse researchers answer questions about data by studying a specific topic and collecting data to answer the question. These data may be numeric, such as scores, and analyzed through statistics, or qualitative data, such as interview transcripts. Both are forms of data to inform a research question. Nurse administrators use data to determine strategic direction and assess performance of a unit, service or division. Nurse leaders of all levels, including national professional organizations such as the American Nurses Association (ANA), use data to define health policy, such as data about safe patient handling bills under review in many states. Data about the numbers of health workers in the United States who are injured on the job by lifting patients, as well as the number of patient injuries caused by being lifted without proper transfer devices were reported at the organizational level, the state level, and the national level to define ANA policies as well as inform pending legislation (ANA, 2015b). ANA directs efforts to improve health through convening professional issues panels that review and revise the publications on the scope and standards of practice for numerous nursing specialties. ANA's Membership Assembly and Professional Issues Panels are charged with setting policy in health care, the workplace, patient care, and many other areas where nurses are engaged. When a hot topic arises or there are various views and opinions about current events, these ANA groups may address these concerns by way of a position statement or resolution on such varied topics of concern to nurses such as bloodborne and airborne diseases, consumer advocacy, substance abuse and ethical considerations. All of these advocacy efforts require various levels of data to influence policy and relevant state and federal regulations.

4

Future Directions in the Use of Quality Data: Electronic Health Records, Telehealth and eMeasures

Digital technology, such as smart phones, tablets, and web-enabled devices, are integral to our daily lives and the way we communicate. Health care has always been an information-rich enterprise and, with the availability of increasingly sophisticated electronic and digital resources, the possibilities for collecting and utilizing data for patient care and organizational efficiencies are expanding exponentially. A greater and more transparent flow of information within a digital healthcare infrastructure, facilitated by electronic health records (EHRs) and other information technologies, demonstrates how digital progress can transform the way care is delivered. With EHRs, information is available whenever and wherever it is needed. In addition to EHRs, other technological innovations, such as telehealth, offer unlimited possibilities in transforming and improving the way health care is provided. The website HealthIT.gov provides up-to-date information on wide range of issues regarding information technology including implementation of government initiatives, impact of policies and research findings.

Healthcare providers, administrators, policy-makers, and payers agree that information technology (IT) has significant potential to improve healthcare quality and safety (IOM, 2001a; US, DHHS, 2010). Collectively referred to as health information technology (HIT), recent projects at the national level focus on advancing the use of EHRs and establishing interoperability standards for health information exchange across institutions (Powner, 2006). Interoperability refers to the extent to which systems and devices can exchange data, and interpret that shared data. This might include exchange of information between different hospitals or between hospitals and other healthcare organizations, such as home care agencies or long-term care facilities. For two systems to be interoperable, they must be able to exchange data and subsequently present that data in a way that can be understood by users at both sides. In other words, an important feature of interoperability is the ability of different information systems to communicate effectively with one another. The implications of widely accepted interoperability among different healthcare organizations on patient outcomes are vast.

The Patient Protection and Affordable Care Act, also known as healthcare reform or Obamacare, contains many provisions regarding the increased use of technological advances such as EHRs, HIT, and health information technology for economic and clinical health (HITECH). This chapter will explore the current and future influence of technological innovations on nursing quality and safety and opportunities for data collection and analysis.

Electronic Health Records and Meaningful Use

According to the government website HealthIT.gov, "an electronic health record (EHR) is a digital version of a patient's paper chart. EHRs are real-time, patient-centered records that make information available instantly and securely to authorized users (US, DHHS, 2015). An EHR system allows the aggregation of patient records to perform a wide range of analytic functions addressing clinical and administrative issues. Among its many functions, EHRs can: (i) serve as repository for documentation of patient's medical history, diagnoses, medications, treatment plans, immunization dates, allergies, radiology images, and laboratory and test results; (ii) allow access to evidence-based tools and decision-support options for patient care, and (iii) automate and streamline provider workflow to increase efficiencies (reduce paperwork; less reliance on handwritten notes) and other process measures.

A review of research literature on EHR (Hayrinen, Saranto, Nykanen, 2008) catalogued the many data components available in EHR including: daily charting, medical administration, admission nursing note, nursing care plan, referral, discharge, and histories, to name a few. The availability of EHR has focused attention on the need for complete and accurate documentation, particularly nursing documentation. Ideally, complete and accurate documentation can facilitate completion of public reporting requirement and monitoring quality measures and outcomes.

One of the most significant benefits of EHR is that the information can be shared with authorized providers within a healthcare organization, as well as potentially across organizations. In this way, all clinicians involved in a patient's care—whether medical specialists, pharmacists, medical imaging, or other provider—can share information with each other and thus reduce duplications, increase care coordination and improve communication. Patients also benefit from EHRs, which often offer patient portals for individuals to be more fully engaged in their care by allowing them to view their medical records and keep in contact with their providers (electronic health records and electronic medical records are used interchangeably).

In addition, utilization of EHR to collect and exchange patient level data increases the overall reliability of the data since similar definitions and measures are used by all participating practitioners. As described in Chapter 2, the availability of reliable quality data is critical to measuring patient and other outcomes.

There is widespread professional agreement regarding the potential value of EHRs, though the cost and resources to successfully implement EHR are significant. To address this obstacle, in 2009 CMS advanced an incentive program to encourage hospitals and physicians offices to adopt EHR. Recent data from the Office of the National Coordinator for Health Information Technology (Charles, Gabriel, & Furukawa, 2014) reports that almost 60% of hospitals have adopted a basic EHR, which includes patient demographics, medication lists, and lab and radiology reports. Approximately one-quarter of the nation's hospitals have adopted comprehensive EHR systems. Taken together, these data represent significant increases in utilization of EHR in acute care settings since 2009 when federal incentives were put in place. The incentive program includes seven stages of adoption and about 37% are in the final three stages of the process (Japsen, 2014). There are variations among the 50 states with regards to EHR adoptions. According to a Data Brief of EHR adoption in 2014, eleven states reported adoption rates below the national average (Charles, Gabriel, & Furukawa, 2014).

There is also the expectation that physician offices and other non-hospital settings will adopt EHR as well (Kokkonen, Davis, Lin, Dabade, Feldman, & Fleischer Jr., 2013). According to a CDC report (Hsiao and Hing, 2014), in 2013, 78% of office-based physicians used some type of EHR, which most typically included electronic billing systems, and 48% have adopted basic systems. A sizable majority (69%) of these private practices report that they plan to take advantage of the meaningful-use incentive plans offered by CMS. Adoption of EHR among physician offices varies by state in a similar fashion to adoption of EHR among hospitals.

In sum, the infusion of fiscal incentives has spurred the growth of EHR in hospitals and physician offices. Adoption of basic EHR is now the norm in most states, though variations do exists. Adoption of comprehensive EHR is growing steadily but stands at 26% in hospitals in 2013.

Both financial and non-financial barriers exist to the adoption of EHR. The cost of purchasing, implementing, and maintaining EHR hardware and software for five physician practices has been estimated $162, 000 plus $85,500 in maintenance fees. In addition, there are costs of implementation teams at the practice as well as systems ends. Moreover, it's estimated that physicians and other clinical and non-clinical staff required on average 134 hours of training (Fleming, Culler, McCorkle, Becker, & Ballard, 2011). In short, despite the clear potential of EHRs for improving quality, safety, and efficiencies, the investment in EHR is too burdensome for many smaller practices and agencies.

As part of the American Recovery and Reinvestment Act of 2009, Congress and the Obama administration provided the healthcare community with a transformational opportunity to support increased use of EHR. The HITECH Act (HITECH) authorized incentive payments through Medicare and Medicaid to clinicians and hospitals when they use EHRs privately and securely to achieve specified improvements in care delivery. Equally important, HITECH's goal is not adoption alone but meaningful use of EHRs—that is, their use by providers to achieve significant improvements in care (Jha, 2010). The legislation ties payments specifically to the achievement of advances in healthcare processes and outcomes (Blumenthal, 2010; Kennedy, Murphy, & Roberts, 2013).

To receive an EHR incentive payment, providers have to demonstrate through specific measures that they are meaningfully using their EHR technology to:

- Improve quality, safety, efficiency, and reduce health disparities
- Engage patients and family
- Improve care coordination, population, and public health
- Maintain privacy and security of patient health information

CMS, which administers the EHR incentive program, has established a timeline for implementation of meaningful use. In Stage 1 (which took place from 2011–2012), provider organizations set up their systems for capturing required data and processes for sharing data internally within their institutions. In this stage, healthcare organizations are expected to meet a set of EHR core objectives such as recording vital signs and chart changes; maintaining current medication records; and providing clinical quality measures to CMS or states, to name a few (Blumenthal, 2010). The expectation of meaningful use incentive program is that, by 2016, recipients of the funding will be able to demonstrate:

- Better clinical outcomes
- Improved population health outcomes
- Increased transparency and efficiency
- Empowered individuals
- More robust research data on health systems

The top three EHR vendors in the country are Cerner, EPIC, and Allscripts (Verdon, 2013). While EHRs have great promise for patient-centered care, and may allow the harvesting of big data, careful design of clinician workflow is key to efficient use of the technology.

Beyond EHR: Computerized Provider Order Entry, Barcodes, and Decision Support Systems

The availability of EHR opened the door to many innovations in health care: computerized provider order entry (CPOE), barcodes, and CDSSs. One of the first applications associated with EHR involved order management which enables providers to electronically order laboratory tests, prescriptions, and other processes. With CPOE, multiple providers can view the order and thereby increase efficiencies and communication among interdisciplinary team members. Most importantly, CPOE systems can eliminate errors occurring at the ordering phase. The potential for CPOE to reduce medication errors and adverse drug events had been recognized as early as the IOM's *Crossing the Quality Chasm: A*

New Health System for the 21st Century in 2001 and a substantial amount of research has been done to assess the outcomes of CPOE systems (Staggers, Weir, & Phansalker in Hughes, 2008).

Whereas CPOE may identify errors at the ordering phase, barcodes are typically used to reduce errors in medication administration phase. Bar coding has been used in multiple ways such as inventory control (as in retail stores, as well as healthcare organizations) and tracking laboratory specimens. However, bar coding allows organizations with EHR to track every phase of the medication process (through scanning the bar), starting with the barcoded wristband given to the patient at admission, to ordering various procedures and tests, to the pharmacist who fills prescriptions and sends medication (also barcoded and boxed) to unit, to the RN checking that the barcoded medicine matches the patient's barcoded wristband. The ultimate goal of the barcode approach is to satisfy the five rights of medication administration—right patient, right drug, right dose, right frequency, and right route (Staggers et al., 2008).

Technological Innovations and Measuring Nursing Quality Processes and Outcomes

In addition to HITECH, the ACA called for the establishment of the *National Quality Strategy* (NQS), which is led by the AHRQ on behalf of the DHHS. The NQS was developed through a collaborative process with input from a range of over 300 stakeholders representing all sectors of the healthcare industry and the general public. Based on this input, the NQS established:

- A set of three overarching aims that builds on the IHI's Triple Aim®
- Supported by six priorities that address the most common health concerns that Americans face
- Using nine levers to align their core business or organizational functions to drive improvement on the aims and priorities (see Sidebar 4.1).

The history and description of the advent and integration of EHR in health care has clear and deep implications to practicing nurses, as well as those engaged in policy, administration, and academia. Nurses have played, and can continue to play important roles in advancing the role of technology to improve the quality and safety of their patients. Nurses have been engaged in many of the governmental advisory committees and workgroups that deliberated the implication of IT, EHR, and meaningful

SIDEBAR 4.1

NATIONAL QUALITY STRATEGY'S AIMS, PRIORITIES AND LEVERS FOR HEALTHCARE QUALITY

The Three Broad Aims

1. **Better Care**: Improve the overall quality by making health care more patient-centered, reliable, accessible, and safe.

2. **Healthy People, Healthy Communities**: Improve the health of the U.S. population by supporting proven interventions to address behavioral, social, and environmental determinants of health in addition to delivering higher-quality care.

3. **Affordable Care**: Reduce the cost of quality health care for individuals, families, employers, and government.

The Six Priorities Set Forth

1. Making care safer by **reducing harm** caused in the delivery of care.

2. Ensuring that **each person and family is engaged** as partners in their care.

3. Promoting effective **communication and coordination** of care.

4. Promoting the most **effective prevention and treatment practices** for the leading causes of mortality, starting with cardiovascular disease.

5. Working with **communities** to promote wide use of best practices to enable healthy living.

6. Making quality care more **affordable** for individuals, families, employers, and governments by developing and spreading National Quality Strategy's healthcare delivery models.

(continued)

NQM's Aims, Priorities and Levers for Healthcare Quality (cont'd)

The Nine NQS Levers

Each of the nine NQS levers represents a core business function, resource, and/or action that stakeholders can use to align to the Strategy.

1. **Measurement and Feedback:** Provide performance feedback to plans and providers to improve care

2. **Public Reporting**: Compare treatment results, costs, and patient experience for consumers

3. **Learning and Technical Assistance:** Foster learning environments that offer training, resources, tools, and guidance to help organizations achieve quality improvement goals

4. **Certification, Accreditation, and Regulation:** Adopt or adhere to approaches to meet quality and safety standards

5. **Consumer Incentives and Benefit Designs**: Help consumers adopt healthy behaviors and make informed decisions

6. **Payment:** Reward and incentivize providers to deliver high-quality, patient-centered care

7. **Health Information Technology:** Improve communication, transparency, and efficiency for better coordinated health and health care

8. **Innovation and Diffusion:** Foster innovation in healthcare quality improvement, and facilitate rapid adoption within and across organizations and communities

9. **Workforce Development:** Investing in people to prepare the next generation of healthcare professionals and support lifelong learning for providers

Source: http://www.ahrq.gov/workingforquality/

use of the nursing practice (Kennedy et al., 2013). Many nursing professional organizations, such as the ANA, have been at the forefront of the policy agenda regarding EHR and HIT.

The American Nurses Association (ANA) has launched and participated in several HIT initiatives (ANA, 2015b):

- Developing standardized nursing languages
- Nominating nurse leaders to federal HIT committees and workgroups
- Developing position statements on HIT initiatives, policy, and standards
- Participating in HIT alliances, including the Alliance for Nursing Informatics, American Medical Informatics Association, Healthcare Information, and Management Systems Society
- Developing educational products that support the consumer eHealth campaign of the Office of the National Coordinator for Health Information Technology
- Coordinating expert panel summit meetings to establish quality measurement models for inclusion in electronic health records

Individual RNs are encouraged to get involved in IT and EHR adoption at their institutions by joining committees that address quality improvement, automated documentation, and patient engagement (Kennedy et al., 2013; ANA, 2009). Some institutions employ nursing informatists who can facilitate communications between IT professional and nursing staff. It is vital that nurses be at the table when decisions about IT and EHR are made since these decisions will most directly impact nursing documentation practices, reporting requirements, and other processes within the nurse's domain. To paraphrase a common adage: nurses have to be part of the decision because these decisions will be made with or without them.

In summary, the work of the NQS and ANA are reminiscent of the landmark IOM reports of 1999, 2001, and 2003 with the focus on patient-centered, technologically inventive approaches to enhancing quality of patient care processes and measurement of patient outcomes. The seemingly slow progress to integrate quality data into the very fabric of health care is testament to the very real and very persistent challenges facing nurses and other providers. Despite almost universal recognition of the long-term positive impact of EHR on patient and practice outcomes, there is still sluggish adoption of EHR and other technological innovations in many sectors of healthcare delivery.

eMeasurement and Nurse-sensitive Indicators

eMeasurement is defined as the secondary use of electronic data to populate standardized performance measures (Dykes & Collins, 2013). eMeasurement is predicated on the availability of electronic systems that contain all the data elements necessary to measure clinical and non-clinical processes and outcomes. eMeasurement goes beyond the presence of an EHR, which focuses primarily on patient care, and includes documentation of the performance of individual nurses and other clinical and non-clinical staff. From the technical point-of-view, data warehousing is a term that computer scientists use to describe the science of storing data for the purpose of meaningful future analysis. A data warehouse enables the electronic storing and retrieving of data so that some analysis can be performed on that data to support a business decision or to predict an outcome. eMeasurement, therefore, would be facilitated and supported by data warehousing. The possibility of analyzing data from different electronic systems within an organization to monitor and measure quality, safety, and other indicators has staggering implications.

Nurse-sensitive performance measures, such as patient falls and hospital-acquired pressure ulcers, have been among first eMeasures to be examined (Dykes & Collins 2013: Wakefield, 2014). Data on falls, for example, may come from different sources (i.e., assessment tools, clinical records, and the incident reporting system). It is possible to bring together information from the different systems to design data reports to meet regulatory requirements, professional accrediting bodies, as well as internal reporting for unit-based and institution-based quality performance and improvement. Given the relatively moderate adoption of EHR and other innovations in settings other than HMOs (health maintenance organizations) and hospitals, there is great potential for discussions and implementation of eMeasurement in the future.

Big Data

Big data is a popular term used to describe the exponential growth and availability of data from many sources. As the name implies, big data refers to the amalgamation of amounts of data so massive that they require newly developed database and software techniques. The uniqueness of big data ability to handle enormous amounts of different types of data at high velocity depends on availability of new IT infrastructures, such as cloud data storage (Roski, Bo-Linn, & Andrews, 2014). Roski and colleagues (2014) sum up the definition of big data as "the three Vs"—volume, variety, and velocity.

In health care, the explosion of electronic health data has resulted in the availability of large amounts of varied patient and provider-level data in digital form. Combining elements of EHRs with claims, census, and population-based data has huge potential for improving patient, financial, and business outcomes. This is the big deal about big data (Weil, 2014).

Big data amplifies the ability to perform more complicated analyzes that have the potential to improve clinical decision-making at the point of care. Tapping into vast databases that go beyond the EHRs, a provider can access data to inform treatment decisions for the individual patient, yielding better decisions and outcomes. Big data also has the potential to revolutionize the way we conduct clinical and health services research, as well as analyses of secondary data (Weil, 2014).

The availability of big data creates enormous opportunities for sophisticated analytic techniques to better understand the confluence of quality and cost. As discussed in an earlier section, there has been a growing interest and demand for predictive modeling and a data-driven assessment tool to improve quality and patient outcomes. Big data has the potential to encourage further precision of analytics, algorithms, and other statistical procedures to assist in clinical and cost-related decision-making in specific areas, such as reducing readmissions and stemming the fiscal impact of high-cost patient populations (Bates, Saria, Ohno-Machado, Shah, & Escobar, 2014). Recent discussion of "high reliability" organizations are predicated on the availability of big data that can be analyzed at great speeds (Chassin, 2011; Riley, Davis, Miller, McCullough, 2010). However, there are many technical, privacy, and data-stewardship issues regarding big data that are still being examined (Roski et al., 2014).

A unique application of big data in an urban setting is the Center for Urban Science and Progress, or CUSP. CUSP, a consortium of world-class universities and prominent international tech companies, was created by NYU Polytechnic School of Engineering as a response to a challenge put forth by New York City to create an applied science campus that would make the city a world capital of science and technology, and dramatically boost its economy. CUSP intends to leverage the vast amounts of data available urban settings to become the world's leading authority in the emerging field of urban informatics—the collection, integration, and analysis of data to understand and improve urban systems and quality of life. (For more information on CUSP see http://cusp.nyu.edu.)

The next section will examine how one state, New York, pioneered investments to encourage the use and sharing of multiple data sources for healthcare decision-making.

States Invest in Health Information: The Case of New York State's HEAL NY programs

Given the huge financial investment necessary to introduce HIT across healthcare delivery settings, different states have provided financial opportunities, grants and incentives to encourage the spread of EHR and interoperability across organizations. New York State passed the Health Care Efficiency and Affordability Law for New Yorkers Capital Grant Program in 2004, often referred to as the HEAL NY Program. New York has identified three dimensions for growth:

1. Increase number and diversity of stakeholders sharing electronic health information
2. Improve the value of participation (improved benefits and reduced costs) through implementation of so-called shared services and coordination with Medicaid HIT efforts
3. Increase the types of information (patient history, labs, medications, etc.) being exchanged

This can be accomplished by determining a level set or minimum floor for information exchange and bringing all participants up to this level (New York eHealth Collaborative, 2009).

HEAL NY represents the largest state-based public investment of its kind, with $250 million worth of grants given to alliances of healthcare stakeholders committed to implementing health information exchange (HIE), interoperable EHRs, electronic prescribing, or some combination of healthcare organizations and regional health information organizations throughout the state (Kern Barron, Abramson, Patel, Kaushal, 2009; Kern, Malhotra, Barron, Quaresimo, Dhopeshwarker, Pchardo, Kaushal, 2013). An evaluation of the early HEAL grant found that 100% of HEAL NY Phase 1 grantees still existed and were attempting to implement interoperable HIT approximately two years after the award announcements. The success of the HEAL-NY was predicated on several factors including the significant financial investment; the strong community involvement in the implementation of the projects and the adoption of a structured approach for building a statewide health information network maximizes a common technical approach (Kern et al., 2009). Moreover, hospitals and other larger provider groups have the capacity to implement HEAL objectives.

Despite its reported success, many impediments remain to interoperability and data exchanges in New York, as well as in other states that have invested in state-wide HIT programs. In addition to the significant financial investments required, reaching desired goals of interoperability and data sharing takes time and requires strong, long-term planning (Kern et al., 2009). One HEAL grant sought to introduce interoperability between the EHR systems in key physician offices and visiting nurse service over a two-year period. The project failed to meet its objectives for a range of reasons including:

- Lack of clearly articulated expectations and timelines for software vendors
- Resistance among physician's offices in adopting EHR and working with software consultants
- Relatively low frequency of referrals between physicians and home care agencies, as compared to relationships with hospitals, to name a few (Rosenfeld, Kim, & Rosati, 2010)

Conceptually, the New York model for health information infrastructure views the different levels of data as building blocks: starting with organizational data at the patient and provider level (e.g., EHR); moving to the clinical level, which is the aggregated data developed by individual organizations to inform decisions, and measure and report organization-specific performance; and finally, the state-wide health information exchanges where all types of healthcare organizations (hospitals, home care, long-term care, etc.) share common data across providers mobilize information for public health and quality reporting (NY eCollaborative, 2009). The successful implementation of the providing interoperability across organization that allows sharing of data is expected to result in improved healthcare quality, reduced costs, and improved outcomes for all New Yorkers.

Future Directions: Telehealth and Personal Digital Assistants

Telehealth, also known as telemedicine, is defined by the DHHS as "the use of technology to deliver health care, health information or health education at a distance" (US, DHHS, 2014).

Telehealth can be divided into two general types of applications: real-time communication, and store-and-forward. Real-time communication may be a patient and a nurse practitioner consulting with a specialist via a live audio-video link, or a physician and a patient in an exam room communicating through an interpreter who is connected by phone or webcam. Store-and-forward refers to the transmission of digital images, as in radiology or dermatology, for a diagnosis. All telehealth applications require HIT, but not every use of HIT can be called telehealth. Stand-alone systems like EHRs or CDSSs are types of HIT that are not typically thought of as telehealth applications. The boundaries of telehealth are limited only by the technology available, and new applications are being invented and tested every day. *Telenursing*—sometimes *telehealth nursing*—refers to the use of such technologies in delivering nursing care and conducting nursing practice from a distance (ATM, 2011).

A literature review conducted by Schlachta-Fairchild, Effrink, and Deickman (2008) identified several telemedicine themes:

1. Diagnosis and teleconsultation

   Diagnoses of disease made through telehealth, for example remote interpretation of electrocardiogram results, has been found to be similar to in-person interpretation (Schwaab et al., 2006). Remote reading of radiologic tests represents another example of the diagnostic potential of telehealth. Similarly, the use of video and computer communication systems (e.g., Skype) makes it possible to provide consultation, patient education, and counseling remotely. Many care coordination and care management programs depend on telephonic communications with patients which may be consider a type of elementary telehealth.

2. Monitoring and surveillance

   A wide variety of telehealth devices have been developed to monitor and track patients remotely. Perhaps the most common application of remote technology for patient care involves medication compliance and adherence devices. Essentially, these digitized pill boxes allow nurses, caregivers, or other providers to determine whether a patient has taken their medication in a timely fashion. These devices are programmed to remind the patient to take their medication and then send electronic communication to a clinician or caregiver if the patient fails to open the pill box and empty its contents after numerous reminders. Ideally, these devices allow patients to self-manage their care and medication adherence and, when necessary, alert clinicians or caregivers when they must step in.

Several popular telehealth devices have been developed for home use with patients with congestive heart failure. With these devices, patients are taught to use a special blood pressure cuff and digital scale at home. The data is electronically sent to a central station and interpreted electronically for abnormalities. If the patient's blood pressure and weight remain within the desired interval, the data is stored on the individual's EHR. However, if there are any changes, the clinician or caregiver is notified to take further action. These sorts of devices have been found to be useful in supplementing home visits from nursing professionals. Hospitals and skilled nursing facilities use telehealth devices for monitoring and surveillance purposes as well. Bed alarms that alert providers that a patient is attempting to get out of bed and alarms placed in patient robes are used to alert staff when a cognitively impaired patient is attempting to leave the unit or building are two common examples.

3. Clinical and health services outcomes

Telemedicine innovations in the area of clinical and health services outcomes are often used to increase communication with patients about their functional and clinical status so that they can take charge of their care. One example is use of mobile phones for patients with diabetes, which are used to help them manage their condition effectively. One diabetes care management program sought to improve self-care management among inner city adolescents with diabetes through a combination of mobile technology, structured clinical education, and support. Cell phones were equipped with mobile application and clinical website portal has enabled the program staff to gather a broad range of data on patients for program evaluation purposes. Preliminary results from the evaluation of the program found minimal engagement among the teenagers, yet statistically significant reductions in HbA1C levels over time (Rosati, Russell, & Ahrens, 2011). However, this evaluation and many others lack sufficient sample sizes or intervention lengths to determine whether the results might be sustained over time. Future research should examine other key issues, such as provider and user perceptions of the devices, integration into a healthcare practice, and cost, which would provide important insight into the use of mobile phones for chronic disease management (Holtz & Lauckner, 2012).

Conclusion

Recent developments in information technologies have radically changed the way patients and clinicians interact. As EHRs and other HIT become more prevalent across the healthcare setting, the opportunities to impact patient outcomes are enormous for individual organizations as well as for interoperable communications across various health entities. The dazzling array of telemedicine and eMeasurement possibilities has the potential to improve efficiencies, standards of care and patient—as well as financial—outcomes. Despite the strong support for EHR and meaningful use among federal and state governments—as well as private and public agencies—significant barriers still remain to universal adoption of HIT and EHR across the healthcare spectrum. Over time, especially in the context of third-party reimbursement and federal government imperatives, the value of exploiting technological innovation in health care will likely be embraced throughout the healthcare system.

5

How Nurses Lead through Data Use and Interpretation: Insights from the Chief Nurse

The power of the nursing profession is driven by our large number and vast knowledge of healthcare delivery, healthcare systems, and our ability to influence directly the outcomes of patients. As the chief nursing officer of a large, urban academic medical center, my role is to ensure that all of the 3,000+ registered nurses and advanced practice nurses understand and act upon their sphere of influence: their patients, their unit, their hospital, their communities. This begins with an understanding of the meaning and importance of data (patient, unit, hospital, community) that reflects the results of the nursing care they deliver each and every day.

There are several examples nationally of how nurses lead quality and safety initiatives and drive change through their use of data. "You manage what you measure" means that to make significant and lasting change, nurses must know their performance data, and understand how to use it to make improvements at the bedside. One of the important competencies of baccalaureate education previously described is nurses improving care. Quality improvement is one of the hallmarks of professional nursing, and it is essential to our patients and our profession that we step up and own our role in improving care at the bedside and all areas where nursing is practiced.

The literature is replete with several studies of nurses using data to improve care outcomes, and all of these studies can be replicated in our practice to further emphasize the critically important role that nurses play in improving the health and safety of the nation (Needleman, Beurhaus, Mattke, Stewart & Zelevinsky, 2002). Improving medication safety (Freeman, McKee, Lee-Lehner, & Peseneker, 2013), improving handoffs at bedside shift reports (Jeffs et al., 2013; Kerr, Lu, & McKinlay, 2013; Sand-Jecklin & Sherman, 2012), and examining shift length (Witkoski Stimpfel & Aiken, 2012) given the popularity of 12-hour shifts in hospital nursing, are all topics that nurses have studied and have contributed greatly to the quality and safety of patient care. All of these studies require nurses to understand the problem, develop a solution, and develop measures (data) to determine if the solution made a difference in patient care.

Nursing's Role in Preventing Hospital-Acquired Conditions

Nurses are essential to the reduction of hospital-acquired conditions (HACs); significant work has been done at our organization to ensure that nurses are full partners in owning their practice at the bedside and participating in interdisciplinary teams to improve care and ensure that we are not harming patients. HACs are tracked by various departments, including clinical quality, nursing quality, and patient safety/risk management, to review selected cases as well as promote organizational learning from those few HACs that do occur. These robust processes require nurses to be at the table to develop these shared solutions, for in today's complex healthcare world, no one discipline can single-handedly ensure quality; it truly does take a village. Our HAC-reduction efforts include a robust interdisciplinary pressure ulcer reduction program, falls reduction programs that include physicians in the post-fall huddles, and treatment plans (Benoit & Mion, 2012). Included below are several examples of unit and patient population data used in our organization for nurses to identify problems and develop solutions to improve care.

For risk reduction of pressure ulcers, a unit report can be run by the nurse manager on any patient with a Braden score indicating that they are at-risk (Braden score <18) (Figure 6). This unit shows one patient at risk, which allows the manager to follow up with the nurse caring for the patient to ensure that care planning addresses this potential patient problem.

IP Patients With Braden Score <=18 [3735039] as of Wed 3/18/2015 2:32 PM

Adm. Room	Adm. Bed	Patient Name/Age/Sex	MRN	Sensory Perceptions	Moisture	Activity	Mobility	Nutrition	Friction and Shear	Braden Score
	01	[redacted] (70 y.o. F)	[redacted]	1->completely limited	4->rarely moist	1->bedfast	1->completely immobile	1->very poor	1->problem	9
	01	(66 y.o. M)		2->very limited	3->occasionally moist	1->bedfast	2->very limited	3->adequate	1->problem	12
	02	[redacted] (32 y.o. F)	[redacted]	4->no impairment	4->rarely moist	1->bedfast	3->slightly limited	3->adequate	3->no apparent problem	18
	01	[redacted] (87 y.o. M)	[redacted]	3->slightly limited	3->occasionally moist	1->bedfast	2->very limited	3->adequate	2->potential problem	14
	01	[redacted] (78 y.o. F)	[redacted]	4->no impairment	3->occasionally moist	2->chairfast	2->very limited	3->adequate	2->potential problem	16

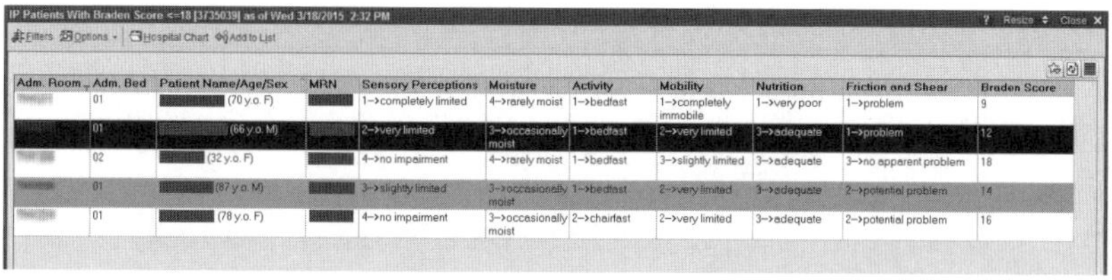

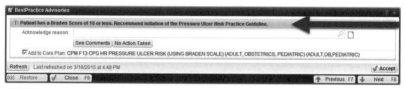

FIGURE 6. **Nurse Manager's Dashboard (Braden Score Indicating At-Risk Patient)**

The "moderate risk" score triggers a Best Practice Alert to add the risk reduction are plan to the patient record (Figure 7).

FIGURE 7. **Best Practice Alert (Braden Score Indicating At-Risk Patient)**

The care plan adds detailed skin assessment documentation to the patient record, which can be reviewed by both the nurse manager and the clinical nurse (Figure 8).

IP Pressure Ulcer Risk Documentation by Dept - Dashboard Use Only [3735312] as of Wed 3/18/2015 4:11 PM

Patient Name/Age/:	MRN	Room and Bed	Braden Score	Braden Q Score	NEONATAL SC	Care Plan Exist	Interventions Dc	Care Plan Type
[redacted] (74 y.o. M)	[redacted]		16			Yes	Yes	Pressure Ulcer Risk
[redacted] (64 y.o. F)	[redacted]		17			No	Yes	
(78 y.o. F)			16			Yes	Yes	Pressure Ulcer
[redacted] (89 y.o. M)	[redacted]		18			No	Yes	
[redacted] (60 y.o. M)	[redacted]		14			Yes	Yes	Pressure Ulcer Risk

[redacted] #[redacted] (CSN: [redacted]) (78 y.o. F) (Adm: 03/08/15)

Skin Assessment

	3/9/2015 0200	3/9/2015 1000	3/9/2015 2230	3/9/2015 2300	3/10/2015 1000	3/10/2015 2200	3/10/2015 2300	3/11/2015 1000
Braden Score (if 18 or less activate Pressure Ulcer, Risk guideline):	17	17	17	17	17	17	17	18
Skin WDL:	ex	WDL	WDL	-	WDL	WDL	-	WDL
Skin Color/Characteristics:	without discoloration	-	consistent with ethnicity	-	consistent with ethnicity	consistent with ethnicity	-	-
Skin Temperature:	warm	warm	warm	-	warm	warm	-	-
Skin Moisture:	dry	dry	dry	-	dry	dry	-	-
Skin Integrity:	rash(es)	-	abrasion(s)	-	abrasion(s)	abrasion(s)	-	abrasion(s)

	3/11/2015 2300	3/12/2015 0900	3/12/2015 2300	3/13/2015 1053	3/13/2015 2300	3/14/2015 1000	3/14/2015 2038	3/15/2015 0900
Braden Score (if 18 or less activate Pressure Ulcer, Risk guideline):	16	16	15	-	15	19	19	19
Skin WDL:	ex	ex	ex	ex	ex	ex	ex	ex
Skin Color/Characteristics:	other (see comments)	other (see comments)	consistent with ethnicity	consistent with ethnicity	consistent with ethnicity	consistent with ethnicity	consistent with ethnicity	consistent with ethnicity
Skin Temperature:	warm	warm	hot	-	warm	warm	warm	warm
Skin Moisture:	moist	moist	moist	-	moist	moist	moist	moist
Skin Integrity:	pressure ulcer(s)	pressure ulcer(s)	-	-	pressure ulcer(s)	pressure ulcer(s)	pressure ulcer(s)	pressure ulcer(s)

	3/15/2015 2200	3/15/2015 2300	3/16/2015 1200	3/16/2015 2300	3/17/2015 0900	3/17/2015 2223	3/17/2015 2300	3/18/2015 0900
Braden Score (if 18 or less activate Pressure Ulcer, Risk guideline):	-	20	16	17	17	-	16	16
Skin WDL:	ex	-	ex	ex	ex	ex	-	ex
Skin Color/Characteristics:	consistent with ethnicity	-	consistent with ethnicity	consistent with ethnicity	consistent with ethnicity	-	-	consistent with ethnicity
Skin Temperature:	warm	-	warm	warm	warm	warm	-	warm

8 of 8 results loaded

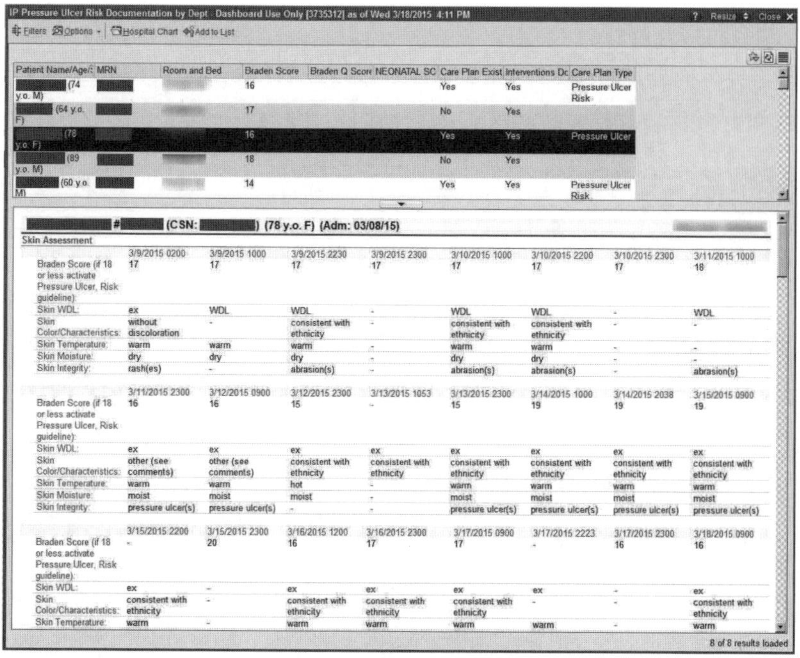

FIGURE 8. **IP Pressure Ulcer Risk Documentation by Department**

In the example below, a unit report is run daily to show any patients at risk for falls (Figure 9). Nurse managers are expected to review with nurses the plan of care that is in place for each patient. The details of the care plan are shown in the bottom of Figure 9.

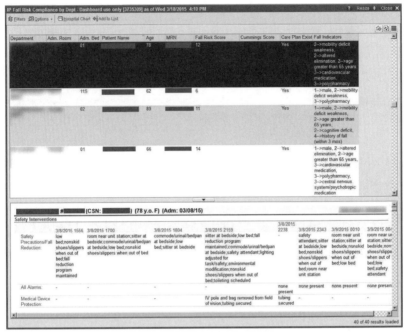

FIGURE 9. **Unit-specific Report for Showing Patients At-Risk for Falls**

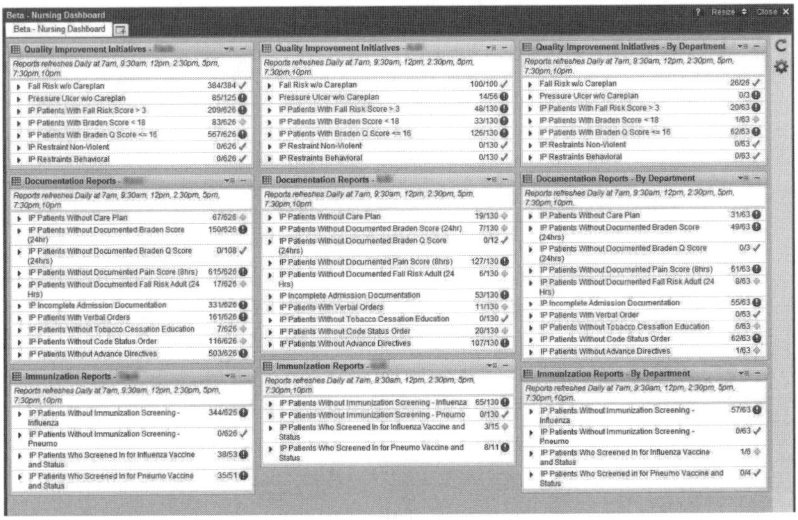

FIGURE 10. **Nurse Manager's Dashboard (All Indicators)**

The nurse manager's dashboard (Figure 10) provides a one-stop view of various quality improvement indicators, elements of the required documentation, and core national reports for nurse managers to monitor their unit's performance. The view for the unit's clinical nurses to monitor their own performance is shown in Figure 11.

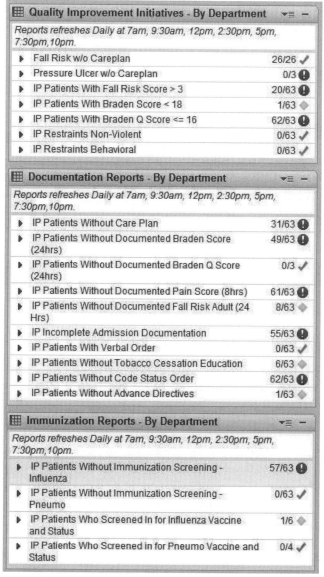

FIGURE 11. Unit Nurse Dashboard

A series of unit-specific report cards are also created to show their trends over time. These reports provide a quarterly view to show performance compared to national benchmarks. (See Appendix A.)

In the perioperative service, tracking the first case offers the care team opportunities to identify ongoing improvements and solutions for troublesome problems.

Several case studies reported in the literature showcase the importance of nurses using data to improve practice with resultant improvement in patient outcomes. While many of these are team-based programs, the changes in practices are often led by nurses. These practice changes include reducing HACs, such as urinary infections and in-hospital falls.

Catheter-Associated Urinary Tract Infections (CAUTI)

Many hospitals are developing strategies to reduce both catheter days (the number of days a patient has an indwelling urinary drainage catheter) and associated infections. If a patient does not have an indwelling urinary catheter, the patient cannot develop a CAUTI. Thus, most interdisciplinary efforts are focused on discontinuing the catheter as soon as possible, as well as adhering to all steps in the guidelines for catheter care for those patients who require an indwelling catheter. Interventions include:

1. Protocol-driven care, where the nurse removes the urinary catheter within 24–48 hours of surgery
2. Standardizing care protocols for the management of the patient with an indwelling catheter
3. Unit-based champions who ensure adherence to care protocols
4. Tracking data in unit-based scorecards (Purvis et al., 2014; Alexaitis & Broome, 2014)

The ANA has been collaborating as a partner with the CMS Partnership for Patients in its quest to reduce HACs. In 2014, a technical expert group convened to develop a streamlined, evidence-based tool for frontline clinicians to use to reduce CAUTIs, as well as create a plan to pilot the tool. ANA plans to make this and other valuable tools available free to frontline RNs on its website. For more information see:

http://nursingworld.org/MainMenuCategories/
ThePracticeofProfessionalNursing/Improving-Your-Practice/
ANA-CAUTI-Reduction-Tool

Falls Prevention

TJC Center for Transforming Healthcare (see http://www.centerfortransforminghealthcare.org) collaborated with seven U.S. hospitals to test a falls prevention program, with a goal of reducing falls by 50%. The methods of robust process improvement tools were used to guide the change management process. TJC's suite of targeted solutions provides standardized interventions proven to assist care teams in reducing falls. Four strategies identified by this study include:

1. Increasing awareness of fall safety across the organization;
2. Empowering patients and families to take an active role in their safety
3. Using a validated falls assessment tool, integrated into an EHR or documentation tools
4. Hourly rounding and patient partnering programs that bring caregivers to the bedside of patients for frequent assessment of those patients determined to be at risk (DuPree, Fritz-Campiz, & Musheno, 2014)

Team training has been demonstrated to reduce falls in one health system (Spiva et al., 2014). Using the TeamSTEPPS model for improving patient safety, team collaboration, and communication among healthcare providers (http://teamstepps.ahrq.gov/), this organization produced a training video for caregivers involved in falls prevention and risk reduction. The team-based intervention program reduced falls by 60% compared to a control group.

Maternity Measures

A major focus on the health of mothers and children, especially at birth, have prompted both government and commercial payers to track maternal health measures such as a reduction in cesarean sections and induced birth before 38 weeks. The World Health Organization Baby-Friendly Hospital Initiative also supports the rights of mothers to choose breastfeeding as their feeding option, and encourages hospitals to develop robust programs to support breastfeeding mothers in hospitals. Since research indicates that mothers who are supported to breastfeed in hospitals do better with breastfeeding at home, many hospitals have signed on to endorse this program. It requires that ten steps of improvement be in place before the Baby-Friendly designation is awarded. NYU Langone became the fourth hospital in New York state, the first academic medical center, and the second hospital in NYC to successfully achieve this designation. Their nurse-led program is illustrative of the power of nurses using data to improve practice.

Care Coordination

Nurses play a major role in care coordination across the continuum, and in preventing readmissions. Patient education efforts to ensure that patients understand their care post-hospitalization are essential in today's hospital environment. The central care delivery model no longer exists, so hospitals must now join with community partners to ensure that patients are safe at home and staying healthy. Post-discharge phone calls, done by nurse care managers at our organization, are one example of how nurses play a central role in keeping patients healthy outside the hospital walls. New roles, such as clinical care coordinators, who manage episodes of care at our organization, use a variety of data sources to monitor the healing progress and long-term health for patients in a CMS bundle-payment demonstration project. These care coordinators may be employed by the hospital or a community health partner, such as the VNSNY.

Magnet Exemplars

Nurses who work in Magnet hospitals are exposed to frequent doses of patient and unit level data. Since Magnet recognition presumes excellence in nursing and patient care, all units must outperform a national benchmark more than half of the time over the four year designation. This demand for excellence is based in the need to review data and address any performance issues. Simply speaking, if you don't have the performance, you are not a Magnet-recognized hospital. Each redesignation requires nurses to raise the bar on their performance and demonstrate continuous improvement. Magnet exemplars describe the structure (policy), the process (an improvement is achieved, such as falls reduction), and the outcome (five or more quarters with improvements against a benchmark). These are clear measures of how a unit's and hospital's care reflect an environment of continuous improvement. Some examples are noted in Table 5.1.

Insights from the CNO: Summary of Key Points

Registered professional nurses are essential to improving the quality of patient care across all healthcare delivery settings. Nurses must have the appropriate knowledge to ensure high-quality care to patients, including

TABLE 5.1. Magnet Hospital Examples of Continuous Quality Improvement

Unit Group (1Q14) Benchmarks (falls rate; with injury rate)	Unit	2013Q4 Reported to NDNQI				2014Q1 Reported to NDNQI				2014Q2 Reported to NDNQI			
		Total Falls		With Injury		Total Falls		With Injury		Total Falls		With Injury	
		#	Rate	#	Rate	#	Rate	#	Rate	#	Rate	#	Rate
Adult Critical Care (1.04; 0.17)	A	0	0.00	0	0.00	1	0.75	0	0.00	2	1.53	0	0.00
	B	1	1.38	0	0.00	1	1.45	1	1.45	0	0.00	0	0.00
	C	3	1.39	0	0.00	6	2.83	0	0.00	4	1.79	2	0.89
Adult Blended Acuity (2.74; 0.53)	D	2	0.86	1	0.43	6	2.58	0	0.00	7	2.97	1	0.42
	E	3	1.95	1	0.65	6	4.57	2	1.52	4	2.85	1	0.71
	17W	7	2.60	2	0.74	6	2.41	0	0.00	2	0.77	0	0.00
	17E	17	7.01	2	0.82	14	5.66	4	1.62	6	2.34	0	0.00
	HCC-11	6	2.79	1	0.46	7	3.39	2	0.97	7	3.15	2	0.90
Adult Step-Down (2.64; 0.49)	14W	1	0.44	1	0.44	2	0.90	1	0.45	2	0.91	1	0.45
	HCC-12	9	6.61	3	2.20	13	9.98	3	2.30	4	3.07	4	3.07
	HCC-13	0	0.00	0	0.00	1	1.63	0	0.00	0	0.00	0	0.00
Adult Surgical (2.55; 0.43)	13E	0	0.00	0	0.00	1	1.19	0	0.00	0	0.00	0	0.00
Adult Moderate Acuity (3.76; 0.54)	11E	2	4.89	0	0.00	0	0.00	0	0.00	3	5.42	0	0.00
	12W	12	6.11	4	2.04	5	2.54	1	0.51	9	4.41	1	0.49
Psychiatry (3.31; 0.75)	HCC-10	6	5.59	3	2.80	4	3.07	3	2.30	3	2.04	0	0.00
Neonatal ICU (0.01; 0.01)	NICU/SCN	0	0.00	0	0.00	0	0.00	0	0.00	0	0.00	0	0.00
Pediatric Critical Care (0.41; 0.08)	PICU	0	0.00	0	0.00	1	1.58	0	0.00	0	0.00	0	0.00
Pediatrics (1.17; 0.35)	CCVCU	0	0.00	0	0.00	0	0.00	0	0.00	1	1.63	0	0.00
	9EAST	1	0.54	0	0.00	3	1.56	0	0.00	2	1.09	1	0.54
Adult Rehab (6.14; 0.68)	HCC-9	13	6.99	2	1.08	10	5.50	2	1.10	8	4.38	2	1.09
Units not reported to NDNQI (benchmark N/A)	13W (Mother)	3	1.07	0	0.00	4	1.50	0	0.00	2	0.73	0	0.00
	16W									1	1.81	1	1.81
OVERALL NYULMC Target: R 2.75; R 2.00		86	2.56	20	0.60	91	2.75	19	0.58	67	1.95	12	0.35

how to identify problems with care, collect relevant data, analyze this data, and develop solutions based on the data. Programs such as Magnet Recognition ensure that healthcare delivery settings support nurses and other relevant disciplines and support staff to achieve the best outcomes for patients. Nurses are involved in hospital and health system governance, and in decision-making for organization-wide purchases, such as information technology systems and new construction.

Nurses play a key role in transitions of care, ensuring that patients' needs are addressed across the continuum of care. New roles for nurses in ambulatory care and in patient-centered medical homes, and new models of community-based care will challenge nurses to look beyond hospitals for new practice settings.

Finally, nursing education must prepare registered professional nurses to practice outside the hospital walls and to lead in new and innovative ways with other health professionals. Nurses, in turn, must embrace these new models of care in the community or within hospitals and be prepared to use their individual and collective voice to improve care for patients in all delivery settings.

Final Thoughts

As the largest workforce of health providers in the nation, registered professional nurses must step up to lead changes in our healthcare delivery system. Developing our voice at the policy and leadership tables requires nurses to improve their levels of knowledge and education in order to be on equal footing with other leaders in healthcare, such as physicians and policy makers. Nurses are viewed by the public as the most trusted professionals, but the least effective at making changes in health care (Gallop, 2015). Recent studies of the nursing workforce suggest that we have to improve our knowledge and participation in hospital quality improvement activities (Djukic et al., 2013). There is great value in harnessing both the numbers and the creativity of registered professional nurses, as staff-led improvements have achieved significant savings of over $600,000 per year per unit (Unruh, Agrawal, & Hassmiller, 2011).

However, our position as the largest group of health professionals will be strengthened by ensuring that all practicing registered nurses are prepared to understand and accept their accountability for ensuring that their patients receive the best care, each and every day, in all delivery settings. Nurses must understand clearly their impact on the health of their patients, and that their nursing care translates to better health for an individual, a group, or a community. Every registered and advanced practice nurse, regardless of educational preparation, must understand and interpret data about their patients to ensure high-quality care. This translates to better outcomes for patients and the public.

APPENDIX A

Unit Report Cards for Clinical Nurses to Improve Practice

These unit-specific report cards were created to show the nurses of a given unit their performance trends over time in addressing HACs (see pages 76-80). These quarterly reports provide a quarterly view to show performance compared to national benchmarks.

Sample Unit Quality Indicators—3Q14

These three figures communicate a quarterly report on patient falls.

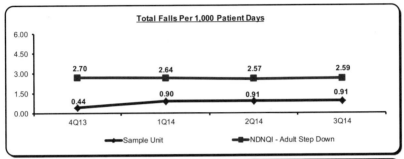

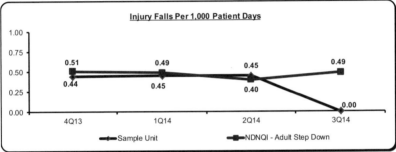

Patient Falls				
	4Q13	1Q14	2Q14	3Q14
Patient Days	2268	2211	2206	2207
# of Patient Falls	1	2	2	2
Minor	1	1	1	0
Moderate	0	0	0	0
Major	0	0	0	0

This pair of figures shows central line infections.

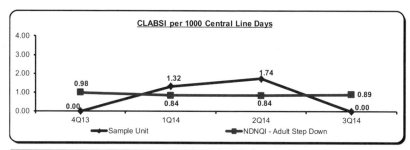

CLABSI								
Sample Unit	4Q13		1Q14		2Q14		3Q14	
	# of CLABS	Line Days	# of CLABS	Line Days	# of CLABS	Line Days	# of CLABS	Line Days
ICU	0	284	1	235	0	155	0	181
Non-ICU	0	524	0	522	1	420	0	401
Total CLABSI	0	808	1	757	1	575	0	582

These two show urinary catheter infections.

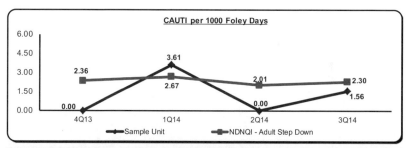

CAUTI								
Sample Unit	4Q13		1Q14		2Q14		3Q14	
	# of CAUTI	Foley Days	# of CAUTI	Foley Days	# of CAUTI	Foley Days	# of CAUTI	Foley Days
ICU	0	152	0	97	0	123	0	148
Non-ICU	0	478	2	457	0	537	1	493
Total CAUTI	0	630	2	554	0	660	1	641

These contain additional metrics that are shared with clinical nurses.

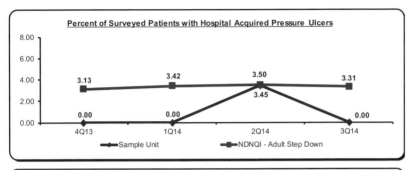

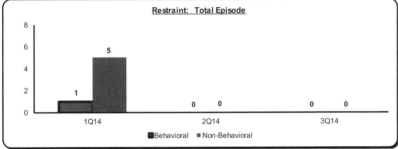

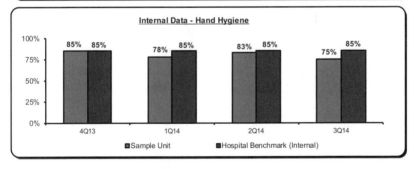

Because this unit is in a Magnet hospital, these three graphs are provided.

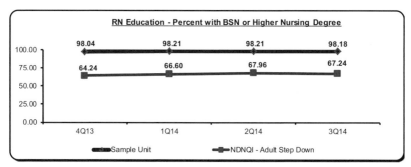

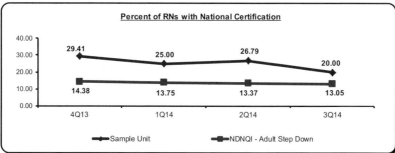

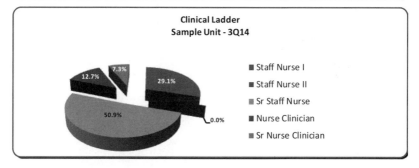

And finally, this table provides the raw data for all the graphed and tabular data displays.

	4Q13	1Q14	2Q14	3Q14
RN Education - Percent with BSN or Higher Nursing Degree				
Sample Unit	98.04	98.21	98.21	98.18
NDNQI - Adult Step Down	64.24	66.60	67.96	67.24
Percent of RNs with National Certification				
Sample Unit	29.41	25.00	26.79	20.00
NDNQI - Adult Step Down	14.38	13.75	13.37	13.05
Total Falls Per 1,000 Patient Days				
Sample Unit	0.44	0.90	0.91	0.91
NDNQI - Adult Step Down	2.70	2.64	2.57	2.59
Injury Falls Per 1,000				
Sample Unit	0.44	0.45	0.45	0.00
NDNQI - Adult Step Down	0.51	0.49	0.40	0.49
Percent of Surveryed Patients with Hospital Acquired Pressure Ulcers				
Sample Unit	0.00	0.00	3.45	0.00
NDNQI - Adult Step Down	3.13	3.42	3.50	3.31
CLABSI Per 1000 Central Line Days				
Sample Unit	0.00	1.32	1.74	0
NDNQI - Adult Step Down	0.98	0.84	0.84	0.89
CAUTI Per 1000 Foley Days				
Sample Unit	0.00	3.61	0.00	1.56
NDNQI - Adult Step Down	2.36	2.67	2.01	2.30
Internal Data - Restraint				
Behavioral		1	0	0
Non-Behavioral		5	0	0
Internal Data - Hand Hygiene				
Sample Unit	85%	78%	83%	75%
Hospital Benchmark (Internal)	85%	85%	85%	85%
Clinical Ladder				
Staff Nurse I	29.09%			
Staff Nurse II	0.00%			
Sr Staff Nurse	50.91%			
Nurse Clinician	12.73%			
Sr Nurse Clinician	7.27%			

REFERENCES

Agency for Healthcare Research and Quality. (2012) *Public reporting as a quality improvement strategy*. Rockville, MD.

Agency for Healthcare Research and Quality. (2013). *Preventing falls in hospitals: A toolkit for improving quality of care*. AHRQ Publication No. 13-0015-EF. Rockville, MD.

Agency for Healthcare Research and Quality. (2015). AHRQuality Indicators. Retrieved from http://www.qualityindicators.ahrq.gov/

Aiken, L. H. (2011). Nurses for the future. *The New England Journal of Medicine, 364*(3), 196–198.

Allan, J. D., & Aldebron, J. (2008). A systematic assessment of strategies to address the nursing faculty shortage. *Nursing Outlook, 56*(6), 286–297.

Alexaitis, I., & Broome, B. (2014). Implementation of a nurse-driven protocol to prevent catheter-associated urinary tract infections. *Journal of Nursing Care Quality, 29*(3), 245–252.

Altman, L. K. (1990, December 5). Heart-surgery death rates decline in New York. *The New York Times*.

American Association of Colleges of Nursing. (2014). The impact of education on nursing practice. Washington, DC: American Association of Colleges of Nursing. Retrieved from http://www.aacn.nche.edu/media-relations/fact-sheets/impact-of-education

American Organization of Nurse Executives. (2005). Practice and education partnership for the future. Washington, DC: American Organization of Nurse Executives.

American Nurses Association. (2008). *Nursing informatics: Scope and standards of practice*. Silver Spring, MD: American Nurses Association.

American Nurses Association. (2009). Position statement on electronic health record. Silver Spring, MD: American Nurses Association. Retrieved from http://nursingworld.org/MainMenuCategories/Policy-Advocacy/Positions-and-Resolutions/ANAPositionStatements/Position-Statements-Alphabetically/Electronic-Health-Record.html

American Nurses Association. (2010). *Nursing: Scope and standards of practice*. Silver Spring, MD: American Nurses Association.

American Nurses Association. (2012). *Nursing's Social Policy Statement: The essence of the profession*. Silver Spring, MD: American Nurses Association.

American Nurses Association. (2015a). Health IT initiatives. Retrieved from http://www.nursingworld.org/MainMenuCategories/ThePracticeofProfessionalNursing/Health-IT

American Nurses Association. (2015b). Professional Issues Panels. Retrieved from http://www.nursingworld.org/MainMenuCategories/Policy-Advocacy/Professional-Issues-Panels

American Nurses Association. Nurse staffing plans & ratios. Retrieved from http://www.nursingworld.org/MainMenuCategories/Policy-Advocacy/State/Legislative-Agenda-Reports/State-StaffingPlansRatios

American Nurses Credentialing Center (2013). *2014 Magnet application manual.* Silver Spring, MD: American Nurse Credentialing Center. Retrieved from http://www.nursecredentialing.org/MagnetApplicationManual

American Telemedicine Association. (2011). Telehealth nursing fact sheet. (ATA Telehealth Nursing SIG.) Washington, DC: Author. Retrieved from http://www.americantelemed.org/docs/default-document-library/fact_sheet_final.pdf?sfvrsn=2

Arthur, J. (2011). *Lean six sigma for hospitals: Simple steps to fast, affordable, and flawless healthcare.* New York: McGraw-Hill Professional.

Bates, D. W., Saria, S., Ohno-Machado, L., Shah, A., & Escobar, G. (2014). Big data in health care: Using analytics to identify and manage high-risk and high-cost patients. *Health Affairs, 33*(7), 1123–1131.

Bekelis, K., Bakhoum, S. F., Desai, A., Mackenzie, T. A., Goodney, P., & Labropoulos, N. (2013). A risk-factor based predictive model of outcomes in carotid endarterectomy: The national surgical quality improvement program 2005–2010. *Stroke, 44*(4), 1085–1090.

Benner, P. (1982). From novice to expert. *The American Journal of Nursing, 82*(3), 402–407.

Benner, P., Sutphen, M., Leonard, V., & Day, L. (2009). *Educating nurses: A call for radical transformation.* San Francisco, CA: Jossey-Bass.

Benoit, R. & Mion, L. (2012). Risk factors for pressure ulcer development in critically ill patients: A conceptual model to guide research. *Research in Nursing & Health, 35*(4), 340–362.

Blumenthal, D. (2010). Launching HITECH. *The New England Journal of Medicine, 362,* 382–385.

Burack, J. H., Impellizzeri, P., Homel, P., & Cunningham, J. N. (1999). Public reporting of surgical mortality: A survey of New York state cardiothoracic surgeons. *The Annals of Thoracic Surgery, 68,* 1195–1200.

Byrnes, J. (2012). Driving value: Solving the issue of data overload with an executive dashboard. *Journal of the Healthcare Financial Management Association, 66*(10), 116–118.

Charles, D., Gabriel, M., & Furukawa, M. (2014). *Adoption of electronic health record systems among U.S. non-federal acute care hospitals: 2008-2013.* ONC Data Brief No. 16. Washington, DC: Office of the National Coordinator for Health Information Technology.

Chassin, M. R. (2002). Achieving and sustaining improved quality: Lessons from New York state and cardiac surgery. *Health Affairs, 21*(4), 40–51.

Chassin, M. R. & Loeb, J. M. (2011). The ongoing quality improvement journey: Next stop, high reliability. *Health Affairs, 30*(4), 559–568.

Chen, L. M., Orav, E. J., & Epstein, A. M. (2012). Public reporting on risk-adjusted mortality after percutaneous coronary interventions in New York state: Forecasting ability and impact on market share and physicians' decisions to discontinue practice. *Circulation Cardiovascular Quality Outcomes, 5*(1), 70–75. doi: 10.1161/CIRCOUTCOMES.111.962761.

Clancy, C. M. (2009, June 11). Patient safety: One decade after *To err is human.* *Patient safety & quality healthcare.* Retrieved from http://psqh.com/ september-october-2009-ahrq

Clarke, S. P., & Aiken, L. H. (2003). Registered nurse staffing and patient and nurse outcomes in hospitals: A commentary. *Policy, Politics, & Nursing Practice, 4*(2), 104–111.

Cronenwett, L. (2012). A national initiative: Quality and safety education for nurses (QSEN). In G. Sherwood, & J. Barnsteiner (Eds.), *Quality and safety in nursing: A competency approach to improving outcomes* (pp. 49–64). Hoboken, NJ: Wiley-Blackwell.

Cronenwett, L., Sherwood, G., & Gelmon, S. B. (2009). Improving quality and safety education: The QSEN learning collaborative. *Nursing Outlook, 57*(6), 304–312.

Davidoff, F., & Batalden, P. (2005). Toward stronger evidence on quality improvement. Draft publication guidelines: The beginning of a consensus project. *Quality and Safety in Health Care, 14*(5), 319–325. doi:10.1136/qshc.2005.014787

De Korne, D. F., van Wijngaarden, J. D., Hiddema, U. F., Bleeker, F. G., Pronovost, P. J., & Klazinga, N. S. (2010). Diffusing aviation innovations in a hospital in the Netherlands. *Joint Commission Journal on Quality and Patient Safety, 36*(8), 339–347.

Djukic, M., Kovner, C. T., Brewer, C. S., Fatehi, F. K., & Seltzer, J. R. (2013). A multi-state assessment of employer-sponsored quality improvement education for early-career registered nurses. *The Journal of Continuing Education in Nursing, 44*(1), 12–19.

Donabedian, A. (1966). Evaluating the quality of medical care. *The Milbank Memorial Fund Quarterly, 44*(3), 166–203.

DuPree, E., Fritz-Campiz, A., & Musheno, D. (2014). A new approach to preventing falls with injuries. *Journal of Nursing Care Quality, 29*(2), 99–102.

Dykes, P. C., & Collins, S. A. (2013). Building linkages between nursing care and improved patient outcomes: The role of health information technology. *The Online Journal of Issues in Nursing, 18*(3), 1–17.

Ellenbecker, C. H., Samia, L., Cushman, M. J., & Alster, K. (2008). Patient safety and quality in home health care. In R. G. Hughes (Ed.), *Patient safety and quality: An evidence-based handbook for nurses.* Rockville, MD: Agency for Healthcare Research and Quality.

Farquhar, M. (2008). *AHRQ quality indicators.* In R.G. Hughes (Ed.), *Patient safety and quality: An evidence-based handbook for nurses.* Rockville, MD: Agency for Healthcare Research and Quality.

Fleming, N. S., Culler, S. D., McCorkle, R., Becker, E. R., & Ballard, D. J. (2011). The financial and nonfinancial costs of implementing electronic health records in primary care practices. *Health Affairs, 30*(3), 481–489.

Foulkes, M. (2011). Nursing metrics: Measuring quality in patient care. *Nursing Standard, 25*(42), 40–45.

Freeman, R., McKee, S., Lee-Lehner, B., & Pesenecker, J. (2013). Reducing interruptions to improve medication safety. *Journal of Nursing Care Quality, 28*(2), 176–185.

Frith, K. H., Anderson, E. F., Caspers, B., Tseng, F., Sanford, K., Hoyt, N. G., & Moore, K. (2010). Effects of nurse staffing on hospital-acquired conditions and length of stay in community hospitals. *Quality Management in Health Care, 19*(2), 147–155.

Gallup. (2014). Honesty/ethics in professions. Retrieved from http://www.gallup.com/poll/1654/honesty-ethics-professions.aspx

Gans, D., Kralewski, J., Hammons, T., & Dowd, B. (2005). Medical groups' adoption of electronic health records and information systems. *Health Affairs, 24*(5), 1323–1333.

Gerhardt, G., Yemane, A., Hickman, P., Oelschlaeger, A., Rollins, E., Brennan, N. (2013). Data shows reduction in Medicare hospital readmission rates during 2012. *Medicare & Medicaid Research Review, 3*(2), E1–E12.

Gray-Miceli, D. (2007). Fall risk assessment for older adults: The Hendrich II fall risk model. *Annals of Long-Term Care, 15*(2). Retrieved from http://www.annalsoflongtermcare.com/article/6786

Griffiths, P., Jones, S., Maben, J., & Murrells, T. (2008). *State of the art metrics for nursing: A rapid appraisal.* London: National Nursing Research Unit, King's College London.

Haberfelde, M., Bedecarré, D., & Buffum, M. (2005). Nurse-sensitive patient outcomes: An annotated bibliography. *Journal of Nursing Administration, 35*(6), 293–299.

Hall, L. M., Doran, D., Laschinger, H. S., Mallette, C., Pedersen, C., & O'Brien-Pallas, L. (2003). A balanced scorecard approach for nursing report card development. *Outcomes Management, 7*(1), 17–22.

Hannan, E. L., Kilburn, H., Jr., O'Donnell, J. F., Lukacik, G., & Shields, E. P. (1990). Adult open heart surgery in New York state: An analysis of risk factors and hospital mortality rates. *Journal of the American Medical Association, 264,* 2768–2774.

Hannan, E. L., Stone, C. C., Biddle, T. L., & DeBuono, B. A. (1997). Public release of cardiac surgery outcomes data in New York: What do NY state cardiologists think about it? *American Heart Journal, 134,* 1120–1128.

Hsiao, C. J., & Hing, E. (2014). Use and characteristics of electronic health record systems among office-based physician practices: United States, 2001–2013. NCHS data brief, no. 143. Hyattsville, MD: National Center for Health Statistics.

Häyrinen, K., Saranto, K., & Nykänen, P. (2008). Definition, structure, content, use and impacts of electronic health records: A review of the research literature. *International Journal of Medical Informatics, 77*(5), 291–304.

Hilton, L. (2012, December 3). BSN in 10 legislation among looming issues for NY/NJ nurses. *Nurse.com.* Retrieved from http://news.nurse.com/article/20121203/NY02/112030021#.U8mS9W3h7XU

Holtz, B., & Lauckner, C. (2012). Diabetes management via mobile phones: A systematic review. *Telemedicine Journal and e-Health, 18*(3), 175–184.

Illich, I. (1975). *Medical nemesis: The expropriation of health.* London: Calder & Boyars.

Institute of Medicine. (1999). *To err is human: Building a safer health system.* Washington, DC: The National Academies Press.

Institute of Medicine. (2001a) *Crossing the quality chasm: A new health system for the 21st century.* Washington, DC.: The National Academies Press (222.ncbi.nlm.nih.gov/books/NBK22857).

Institute of Medicine. (2001b). *Improving the quality of long-term care.* Washington, DC: The National Academies Press.

Institute of Medicine. (2003). *Health professions education: A bridge to quality.* Washington, DC: The National Academies Press.

Institute of Medicine. (2004). *Keeping patients safe: Transforming the work environment of nurses.* Washington, DC: The National Academies Press. (222.ncbi.nlm. nih.gov/books/NBK22857)

Institute of Medicine. (2010). *The future of nursing: Leading change, advancing health.* Washington, DC: The National Academies Press.

Japsen, B. (2014). Despite stimulus dollars, hundreds of hospitals still use mostly paper records. Retrieved from http://www.forbes.com/sites/brucejapsen/2014/03/29/despite-stimulus-dollars-hundreds-of-hospitals-still-use-mostly-paper-records/

Jeffs, L., Acott, A., Simpson, E., Campbell, H., Irwin, T., Lo, J., & Cardoso, R. (2013). The value of bedside shift reporting: Enhancing nurse surveillance, accountability, and patient safety. *Journal of Nursing Care Quality, 28*(3), 226–232.

Jha, A. K. (2010). Meaningful use of electronic health records: The road ahead. *Journal of the American Medical Association, 304*(15), 1709–1710.

The Joint Commission. (2015). National patient safety goals. Oakbrook Terrace, IL: Joint Commission Resources. Retrieved from http://www.jointcommission.org/standards_information/npsgs.aspx

Kansagara, D., Englander, H., Salanitro, A., Kagen, D., Theobald, C., & Kripalani, S. (2011). Risk prediction models for hospital readmission: A systematic review. *Journal of the American Medical Association, 306*, 1688–1698. Report prepared for Veterans Health Administration, U.S. Department of Veteran Affairs.

Kaplan, R. S. & Norton, D. P. (1996). *The balanced scorecard: Translating strategy into action.* Boston: Harvard Business School Press.

Kendall-Gallagher, D., Aiken, L. H., Sloane, D. M., & Cimiotti, J. P. (2011). Nurse specialty certification, inpatient mortality, and failure to rescue. *Journal of Nursing Scholarship, 43*(2), 188–194.

Kennedy, R., Murphy, J., & Roberts, D. W. (2013). An overview of the National Quality Strategy: Where do nurses fit? *The Online Journal of Issues in Nursing, 18*(3), 1–11.

Kenney, C. (2010). *Transforming health care: Virginia Mason Medical Center's pursuit of the perfect patient experience.* Boca Raton, FL: CRC Press.

Kerr, D., Lu, S., & McKinlay, L. (2013). Bedside handover enhances completion of nursing care and documentation. *Journal of Nursing Care Quality, 28*(3), 217–225.

Kern, L. M., Barrón, Y., Abramson, E. L., Patel, V., & Kaushal, R. HEAL NY: Promoting interoperable health information technology in New York state. *Health Affairs, 28*(2), 493–504.

Kern, L. M., Malhotra, S., Barrón, Y., Quaresimo, J., Dhopeshwarkar, R., Pichardo, M., & Kaushal, R. (2013). Accuracy of electronically reported "Meaningful Use" clinical quality measures. *Annals of Internal Medicine, 158*, 77–83.

Kokkonen, E. W., Davis, S. A., Lin, H. C., Dabade, T. S., Feldman, S. R., & Fleischer, A. B., Jr. (2013). Use of electronic health records differs by specialty and office settings. *Journal of the American Medical Informatics Association, 20*(1), 33–38.

Kovner, C. & Gergen, P. J. (1998). Nurse staffing levels and adverse events following surgery in U.S. hospitals. *Image-Journal of Nursing Scholarship, 30*(4), 315–321.

Kurtzman, E., & Fauteux, N. (2014, March). Ten years after "Keeping patients safe": Have nurses' work environments been transformed? *Charting Nursing's Future*, (22).

Lansky, D. (2012, April 9). Public reporting of health care quality: Principles for moving forward [blog post]. Retrieved from http://healthaffairs.org/blog/2012/04/09/public-reporting-of-health-care-quality-principles-for-moving-forward/

Lee, J., Cain, C., Young, S., Chockley, N., & Burstin, H. (2005). The adoption gap: Health information technology in small physician practices. *Health Affairs, 24*(5), 1364–1366.

Lucero, R. J., Lake, E. T., & Aiken, L. H. (2010). Nursing care quality and adverse events in U.S. hospitals. *Journal of Clinical Nursing, 19*(15-16), 2185–2195.

Maas, M., Johnson, M., & Moorhead, S. (1996). Classifying nursing-sensitive patient outcomes. *Image: Journal of Nursing Scholarship, 28*(4), 295–301.

McClure, M. L., Poulin, M. A., Sovie, M. D., & Wandelt, M. A. (1983). *Magnet hospitals: Attraction and retention of professional nurses*. Kansas City, MO: American Nurses Association.

McHugh, M. D., & Witkoski Stimpfel, A. (2012). Nurse reported quality of care: A measure of hospital quality. *Research in Nursing & Health, 35*(6), 566–575.

McHugh, M. D., Berez, J., & Small, D. S. (2013). Hospitals with higher nurse staffing had lower odds of readmissions penalties than hospitals with lower staffing. *Health Affairs, 32*(10), 1740–1747.

McNeill, D. (2013). *A framework for applying analytics in healthcare: What can be learned from the best practices in retail, banking, politics, and sports*. Upper Saddle River, NJ: FT Press.

Melnyk, B. M., Fineout-Overholt, E., Gallagher-Ford, L., & Kaplan, L. (2012). The state of evidence-based practice in U.S. nurses: Critical implications for nurse leaders and educators. *Journal of Nursing Administration, 42*(9), 410–417.

Mick, J. (2011). Data-driven decision making: A nursing research and evidence-based practice dashboard. *Journal of Nursing Administration, 41*(10), 391–393.

Mitchell, P. H. (2008). Defining patient safety and quality care. In R. G. Hughes (Ed.), *Patient safety and quality: An evidence-based handbook for nurses*. Rockville, MD: Agency for Healthcare Research and Quality.

Morse, J. M., Tyylko, S. J. (1989). Development of a scale to identify the fall-prone patient. *Canadian Journal on Aging, 8*(4), 366–377.

National Advisory Council on Nurse Education and Practice. (2010). *The impact of the nursing faculty shortage on nurse education and practice*. Ninth annual report to the Secretary of the U.S. Department of Health and Human Services and the U.S. Congress. Washington, DC: National Advisory Council on Nurse Education and Practice.

National Quality Forum. (2015). Retrieved from http://www.qualityforum.org/story/About_Us.aspx

Naylor, M. D., Lustig, A., Kelley, H. J., Volpe, E. M., Melichar, L., & Pauly, M. V. (2013). The interdisciplinary nursing quality research initiative. *Medical Care, 51*(4), S6–14.

New York City Health. (2013). Making breastfeeding the norm: A report on breastfeeding rates and supportive practices in New York City birth hospitals. Retrieved from http://www.nyc.gov/html/doh/downloads/pdf/ms/breastfeeding-rates-report.pdf

New York State Assembly (2015). Bill A03945 summary. Albany, NY: New York State Legislature. Retrieved from https://legiscan.com/NY/text/A03945/id/1099445/New_York-2015-A03945-Introduced.html

New York eHealth Collaborative. (2009). State HIE cooperative agreement program strategic plan: Achieving meaningful use of health information in New York. NY: New York eHealth Collaborative. Retrieved from https://www.health.ny.gov/funding/rfa/inactive/0903160302/health_it_strategic_plan.pdf

Needleman, J., Buerhaus, P., Mattke, S., Stewart, M., & Zelevinsky, K. (2002). Nurse-staffing levels and the quality of care in hospitals. *The New England Journal of Medicine, 346*(22), 1715–1722.

Needleman, J., Buerhaus, P., Pankratz, V. S., Leibson, C. L., Stevens, S. R., & Harris, M. (2011). Nurse staffing and inpatient hospital mortality. *The New England Journal of Medicine, 364*(11), 1037–1045.

Page, A. E. K. (2008). Practice implications of keeping patients safe. In R. G. Hughes (Ed.), *Patient safety and quality: An evidence-based handbook for nurses.* Rockville, MD: Agency for Healthcare Research and Quality.

PatientCareLink. Retrieved from http://www.patientcarelink.org/about-patientcarelink.aspx

Powner, D. A. (2006). *Health information technology: HHS is continuing efforts to define a national strategy.* Washington, DC: Statement for the United States Government Accountability Office.

Pronovost, P. J., Goeschel, C. A., Olsen, K. L., Pham, J. C., Miller, M. R., Berenholtz, S. M., Clancy, C. M. (2009). Reducing health care hazards: Lessons from the commercial aviation safety team. *Health Affairs, 28*(3), 479–489.

Purvis, S., Gion, T., Kennedy, G., Rees, S., Safdar, N., VanDenBergh, S., Weber, J. (2014). Catheter-associated urinary tract infection: A successful prevention effort employing a multipronged initiative at an academic medical center. *Journal of Nursing Care Quality, 29*(2), 141–148.

Riley, W., Davis, S. E., Miller, K. K. & McCullough, M. (2010). A model for developing high-reliability teams. *Journal of Nursing Management, 18*(5), 556–563.

Robert Woods Johnson Foundation. (2009). *To err is human: Ten years later.* Retrieved from http://www.inqri.org/sites/default/files/TenYrsLater%20FINAL.pdf

Rosati, R. J. (2009). History of quality measurement in home health care. *Clinics in Geriatric Medicine, 25*(1), 121–134.

Rosati, R. J. & Huang, L. (2007). Development and testing of an analytic model to identify home healthcare patients at risks for a hospitalization within the first 60 days of care. *Home Health Care Services Quarterly, 26*(4), 21–36.

Rosati, R. J., Russell, D., & Ahrens, J. (2011). *Using mobile technology to enhance pediatric diabetes care management.* Paper presented at the Third International Conference on eHealth, Telemedicine, and Social Medicine of eTELEMED, Gosier, France.

Rosenfeld, P. (2006). Measurement. In E. A. Capezuti, M. L. Malone, P. R. Katz, & M. D. Mezey (Eds.), *The Encyclopedia of Elder Care* (Vol. 2). New York: Springer.

Rosenfeld, P., Kim, C., & Rosati, R. J. (2010). *Evaluating the outcomes of New York Community Home Health Care Interoperability Program (NYCHHIP): Understanding the challenges of evaluating technological innovations in home care.* Paper presented at the Annual Research Meeting (ARM) of AcademyHealth, Boston, MA.

Roski, J., Bo-Linn, G. W., & Andrews, T. A. (2014). Creating value in health care through big data: Opportunities and policy implications. *Health Affairs, 33*(7), 1115–1122.

Russell, D., Rosenfeld, P., Ames, S., & Rosati, R. J. (2010). Using technology to enhance the quality of home health care: Three case studies of health information technology initiatives at the Visiting Nurses Service of New York. *Journal for Healthcare Quality, 32*(5), 22–29.

Ryan, A. M., Nallamothu, B. K., & Dimick, J. B. (2012). Medicare's public reporting initiative on hospital quality had modest or no impact on mortality from three key conditions. *Health Affairs, 31*(3), 585–592.

Sand-Jecklin, K., & Sherman, J. (2012). Incorporating bedside report into nursing handoff: Evaluation of change in practice. *Journal of Nursing Care Quality, 28*(2), 186–194.

Savitz, L. A., Jones, C. B., & Bernard, S. (2005). Quality indicators sensitive to nurse staffing in acute care settings. In K. Henriksen, J. B. Battles, E. S. Marks, & D. I. Lewin (Eds.), *Advances in patient safety: From research to implementation* (Vol. 4). Rockville, MD: Agency for Healthcare Research and Quality.

Schlachta-Fairchild, L., Effrink, V., & Deickman, K. (2008). Patient safety, telenursing, telehealth. In R. G. Hughes (Ed.), *Patient safety and quality: An evidence-based handbook for nurses.* Rockville, MD: Agency for Healthcare Research and Quality.

Schwaab, B., Katalinic, A., Richardt, G., Kurowski, V., Krüger, D., Mortensen, K., Lorenz, E., & Sheikhzadeh, A. (2006). Validation of 12-lead tele-electrocardiogram transmission in the real-life scenario of acute coronary syndrome. *Journal of Telemedicine and Telecare, 12*(6), 315–318.

Shekelle, P. G. (2013). Quality indicators and performance measures: Methods for development need more standardization. *Journal of Clinical Epidemiology, 66*(12), 1338–1339.

Sim, I., Gorman, P., Greenes, R. A., Haynes, R. B., Kaplan, B., Lehmann, H., & Tang, P. C. (2001). Clinical decision support systems for the practice of evidence-based medicine. *Journal of the American Medical Informatics Association, 8*(6), 527–534.

Sloane Donaldson, M. (2008). An overview of *To err is human*—Reemphasizing the message of patient safety. In R. G. Hughes (Ed.), *Patient safety and quality: An evidence-based handbook for nurses.* Rockville, MD: Agency for Healthcare Research and Quality.

Smith, H. L. (2013). Public Reporting of Medicare Quality Data. *PT in Motion, 5*(10), 44.

Spetz, J., Bates, T., Chu, L., Lin, J., Fishman, N. W., & Melichar, L. (2013). Creating a dashboard to track progress toward IOM recommendations for the future of nursing. *Policy, Politics, & Nursing Practice, 14*(3-4), 117–124.

Spiva, L., Robertson, B., Delk, M. L., Patrick, S., Kimrey, M. M., Green, B., & Gallagher, E. (2014). Effectiveness of team training on fall prevention. *Journal of Nursing Care Quality, 29*(2), 164–173.

Staggers, N., Weir, C., & Phansalkar, S. (2008). Patient safety and health information technology: Role of the electronic health record. In R. G. Hughes (Ed.), *Patient safety and quality: An evidence-based handbook for nurses.* Rockville, MD: Agency for Healthcare Research and Quality.

Unruh, L., Agrawal, M., & Hassmiller, S. (2011). The business case for transforming care at the bedside among the "TCAB 10" and lessons learned. *Nursing Administration Quarterly, 35*(2), 97–109.

U.S. Department of Health and Human Services, Health Resources and Services Administration. (2015). Retrieved from HealthIT.gov

U.S. Department of Health and Human Services, Health Resources and Services Administration. (2014). The future of the nursing workforce: National-and state-level projections, 2012–2025. Retrieved from http://bhpr.hrsa.gov/healthworkforce/supplydemand/nursing/workforceprojections/index.html

U.S. Department of Health and Human Services, Health Resources and Services Administration. (2006). Physician supply and demand: Projections to 2020. Retrieved from http://bhpr.hrsa.gov/healthworkforce/supplydemand/medicine/physician2020projections.pdf

U.S. Department of Health and Human Services, Health Resources and Services Administration. (2010). The registered nurse population: Findings from the 2008 national sample survey of registered nurses. Retrieved from http://bhpr.hrsa.gov/healthworkforce/rnsurveys/rnsurveyfinal.pdf

U.S. Department of Health and Human Services, Health Resources and Service Administration. (2014). What is telehealth? Retrieved from http://www.hrsa.gov/healthit/toolbox/RuralHealthITtoolbox/Telehealth/whatistelehealth.html

U.S. Department of Labor, Bureau of Labor Statistics. (2013, May). Occupational employment and wages: 29-1141 registered nurses. Retrieved from http://www.bls.gov/oes/current/oes291141.htm

Verdon, D. R. (2013). Exclusive report: Top 100 EHRs. *Medical Economics, 90*(20), 19–25.

Wakefield, B. J. (2014, May). The eHealth Measures Compendium. *U.S. Department of Veterans Affairs Forum.* Retrieved from http://www.hsrd.research.va.gov/publications/forum/may14/default.cfm?ForumMenu=may14-3

Wakefield, M. K. (2008). The quality chasm series: Implications for nursing. In R. G. Hughes, (Ed.), *Patient safety and quality: An evidence-based handbook for nurses.* Rockville, MD: Agency for Healthcare Research and Quality.

Weil, A. R. (2014). Big data in health: A new era for research and patient health. *Health Affairs, 33*(7), 1110.

Werner, R. M. & Bradlow, E. T. (2010). Public reporting on hospital process improvements is linked to better patient outcomes. *Health Affairs, 29*(7), 1319–1324.

Wilf-Miron, R., Lewenhoff, I., Benyamini, Z., & Aviram, A. (2003). From aviation to medicine: Applying concepts of aviation safety to risk management in ambulatory care. *Quality & Safety in Health Care, 12*(1), 35–39.

Witkoski Stimpfel, A. & Aiken, L. H. (2012). Hospital staff nurses' shift length associated with safety and quality of care. *Journal of Nursing Care Quality, 28*(2), 122–129.

INDEX